A volume in the series
The Culture and Politics of Health Care Work

Edited by Suzanne Gordon and Sioban Nelson

For a list of books in the series, visit our website at cornellpress.cornell.edu

HELPING SOLDIERS HEAL

How the US Army Created a Learning Mental Health Care System

Jayakanth Srinivasan
Christopher Ivany

ILR PRESS

AN IMPRINT OF CORNELL UNIVERSITY PRESS ITHACA AND LONDON

First published 2021 by Cornell University Press

Printed in the United States of America

Library of Congress Cataloging-in-Publication Data

Names: Srinivasan, Jayakanth, author. | Ivany, Christopher, 1975– author.
Title: Helping soldiers heal: how the US Army created a learning mental health care system / Jayakanth Srinivasan, Christopher Ivany.
Description: Ithaca, [New York]: ILR Press, an imprint of Cornell University Press, 2021. | Series: The culture and politics of health care work | Includes bibliographical references and index.
Identifiers: LCCN 2021005658 (print) | LCCN 2021005659 (ebook) | ISBN 9781501760501 (hardcover) | ISBN 9781501760525 (pdf) | ISBN 9781501760518 (epub)
Subjects: LCSH: Soldiers—Mental health services—United States. | United States—Armed Forces—Mental health services.
Classification: LCC UH629.3 .S85 2021 (print) | LCC UH629.3 (ebook) | DDC 355.3/45—dc23
LC record available at https://lccn.loc.gov/2021005658
LC ebook record available at https://lccn.loc.gov/2021005659

Contents

Acknowledgments

This book tells the story of the Army's transformation into a learning mental health care system, a journey possible only because of the tireless dedication of behavioral health clinicians and the courage of soldiers and their families. In the end, it comes down to clinicians and patients working together to solve problems.

We would like to thank General Peter Chiarelli (retired) and General James C. McConville, who provided support and guidance throughout the transformation. Lieutenant General Patricia Horoho (retired), the 43rd Army surgeon general, set the vision of the Army's operating company model and empowered the Army team to translate her vision into action. Lieutenant General Howard Bromberg (retired) and Lieutenant General Joseph Anderson (retired) pushed us to incorporate the operational perspective and to remember the "true north" of improving the lives of soldiers and their families.

We would like to thank Dr. Jonathan Woodson, who as the assistant secretary of defense for health affairs drove us to understand truly the experience of care and to use data to support our observations. He was instrumental in creating the Department of Defense's policy architecture for measurement-based care. Dr. Michael Dineen pushed us to think big, see the truth, and use policy to create change.

We want to thank the Army's Behavioral Health leadership team. Colonel Millard Brown, the principal force behind the Army's transition to measurement-based care, spent countless hours educating and arguing with us. Colonel Samuel Preston and Colonel Dennis Sarmiento are not only incredible clinicians, but also great soldiers and teachers; they continue to improve the Army's behavioral health system. Command Sergeant Major Ron Dean (retired) taught us how real change happens in the Army, unafraid of ruffling a few feathers along the way. Drs. Kay Beaulieu, Doris Lancaster, and Kelly Moss formed the first Embedded Behavioral Health leadership team at Fort Carson and, by doing so, launched it on an unprecedented scale. Colonel Fred Reeves (retired) saw the impact of behavioral health care transformation on other parts of the Army's resilience framework and pushed to expand the learning across the Army. Among many other accomplishments, Colonel David Orman (retired) and Lieutenant Colonel Ed Brusher (retired) had the vision to build a leadership team well before anyone else even saw the need for one. Colonel Charles Hoge (retired) was the unflappable voice of the scientific literature. He kept all the changes grounded in what could be proven to help the soldier. Thank you all.

JK would like to thank several people specifically. The MIT Army team supported the research. Prof. John Carroll, Prof. Debbie Nightingale, and Dr. Tenley Albright were sounding boards that helped me rethink what practice-based research should be. Andrea Ippolito, John Hess, Lieutenant Colonel Shane Scott, Dr. Dhaval Adojha, Dmitry Lyan, Dr. Armen Mkrtychyan, and Prof. Julia DiBenigno traveled all over the world and learned the Army with me. I also thank my family for the love and support you have always given me. My parents Shri K. Srinivasan and Smt. Bhuvaneswari Srinivasan set the foundation for doing work that matters. My children Veylan and Kartik were born during this project and grew up hearing Army stories. My better half Neira—you are the reason I could be in the field while you kept everything together on the homefront. You and the kids make me a better person every day.

Chris would like to specifically thank several people. Colonel Peyton Hurt (retired) encouraged me to figure out what I really believed in. My parents Major General Robert Ivany (retired) and Marianne Ivany showed me how selfless leaders take care of soldiers and their families. My siblings Mark, Julianne, and Brian (and now Joe and Debra), selfless leaders in their own right, inspire me every day. My children Rachel, Nick, and Ethan have supported me throughout my career and bring fun to every endeavor. My wife Buffy has been my loving and unwavering partner through it all. The best physician in the family, she is—more importantly—the center of our family.

Finally, we would like to thank Scott Cooper, our editor, who demonstrated extraordinary patience, creativity, and skill, and managed to blend our voices to tell one story.

HELPING SOLDIERS HEAL

INTRODUCTION

On September 29, 2010, Admiral Mike Mullen, the chairman of the Joint Chiefs of Staff, the highest-ranking military advisor to the US president, convened a meeting with senior leaders from each of the armed services in the "tank"—his conference room at the Pentagon. In the preceding months, Mullen had grown increasingly concerned about the mental health of those serving in the armed forces and wanted a fresh look at the problem. He had heard about intriguing work Dr. Tenley Albright, the director of the Massachusetts Institute of Technology (MIT) Collaborative Initiatives, had done to examine how systems of care worked for those who had suffered strokes, and he wanted to take a similar approach to military mental health care.[1] MIT's Lean Advancement Initiative—where one of the present authors, Dr. Jayakanth Srinivasan (JK), was then a lead researcher—had done extensive research on enterprise transformation, and they signed on with Dr. Albright to analyze the military's system. Admiral Mullen introduced the MIT team and kicked off the project.

The team spent the first six months of the project researching the publicly available reports, policies, and academic papers related to military mental health care and talking to people with stars on their shoulders—generals and admirals—and senior civil servants in and around the Pentagon. Those conversations surfaced several recurrent themes: military hospitals could not support the new level of demand for mental health care services; there were not enough clinicians to meet the needs of service members and their families; existing data systems did not provide meaningful information about mental health care; clinics were organized around providers, not patients; and the military had no way to assess the actual quality of care it was providing. These insights also strongly mirrored public reports such as that of the Department of Defense (DoD) Task Force on Mental Health and the RAND report on quality of mental health care.[2] The military leadership seemed to know the problems, but they remained unsolved. The project team wondered why.

In parallel, project members had hoped to visit military treatment facilities, which provided much of the mental health care. Admiral Mullen had written a letter of introduction asking the Army, Navy, Air Force, and Marine Corps to support the researchers, which the team—following the required protocol—had sent along to the appropriate offices. But it was not leading to responses and opportunities to visit.

The following May, Dr. Jonathan Woodson, the assistant secretary of defense for health affairs and senior leader in charge of the military health system, asked for an update on the project. The MIT team delivered to him a detailed presentation of the findings from the literature review and the interviews with senior leaders. Woodson flipped through the slides. "We know all these themes! What is actually going on in military treatment facilities?" No one on the team had yet visited a single military installation. Hearing that, Woodson thanked the team for their time and walked out of the room. It was fifteen minutes into a meeting scheduled for an hour.

Woodson's rebuke was stunning. The brief had simply reiterated that the military health system was broken, but offered no new insights as to the reasons why, or any recommendations to fix it. The team had done what numerous consultants and "experts" had done before—offered a superficial analysis to senior DoD leaders that did not reflect the lived experience of care providers, leaders, or health care users. To truly help the military health system change, the team needed to understand what was actually happening in military treatment facilities. That would require an entirely new approach—one that examined behavioral health care in the military from the inside out and from the bottom up.

In 2011, the Army, Navy, and Air Force operated distinct health care systems (the Marines receive medical support from the Navy), each with a different approach to organizing and delivering mental health care, so the MIT team partitioned the study by service branch and JK took on the Army portion of the study. The Army has the largest burden of psychological health injuries among all the service branches.

JK set out to identify the root causes underlying the inability of individual Army hospitals to deliver the needed mental health care and work with the Army to address them. Only talking to the people involved in mental health care could do the former; the latter would require establishing collaborative working relationships with the people who were trying to change it for the better.

At the kickoff meeting in the "tank" months earlier, General Peter Chiarelli, the Army vice chief of staff, had promised to intervene if MIT researchers faced any hurdles when arranging visits to Army installations. He had told JK to reach out directly if there were problems gaining access. Having followed all the required protocols to get access to sites, and not making any progress, JK emailed General Chiarelli and asked for help. Soon after, JK received a call from Dr. Kathleen Quinkert, General Chiarelli's special assistant.

"The Vice asked me to work with you to get the visits set up," she said. "Where do you want to go? When can you leave? Who do you need to talk to?"

JK requested access to at least six Army posts that deployed large numbers of soldiers to Iraq and Afghanistan.[3] The MIT team wanted to determine whether there was variation in how medical treatment facilities provided mental health services to soldiers and their families. With Dr. Quinkert's intervention, JK and four of his graduate students visited Army installations across the country, from Walter Reed Army Medical Center in Washington, D.C., to Tripler Army Medical Center in Hawaii, between July and September 2011. (It came as little surprise when the Hawaii facility was the only place where all the graduate students volunteered to collect data.)

In each visit, the MIT researchers traced the steps soldiers and their families actually took to access mental health care services. They spoke with clinicians, case managers, front desk staff, commanders, chaplains, personnel at other support agencies (such as the substance abuse and suicide prevention offices), military treatment facility leaders, and other senior leaders—including generals and their staffs. During each seven-day visit, the MIT team spoke with more than one hundred people.

From the visits, it became clear that each Army hospital delivered different care in different ways. One hospital's primary approach was group therapy; another relied on individual appointments. One hospital emphasized alternative approaches such as meditation and yoga, while another offered only traditional psychotherapies with relatively strong links to evidence of their effectiveness in recent trials. By talking to and observing people on each post, the MIT researchers began to understand the rationale for these differences, which were sometimes based on the preferences of the providers in leadership positions, opinions of the line commanders assigned there at the time, and even advice from nonexperts. In other places, the MIT team discovered clinical programs based on innovative ideas and designed around real problems facing soldiers with behavioral health problems. Those solutions tended to be more effective and were probably worthy of being implemented across the Army, but no one else—especially leaders back in Washington—seemed to know much about them.

What was very clear was that the Army lacked an Army-wide system of care that soldiers and their families could count on to deliver, no matter where they might find themselves assigned, let alone a health care system that continually learned and improved its performance. It was an "organized anarchy," the result of reactive evolution as each hospital tried independently to address the needs of its local population.[4] Unfortunately, the team frequently encountered disappointed patients, unhappy commanders, and frustrated clinicians.

Fort Carson, Colorado, was one of those first six locations to which members of the MIT team traveled. There, JK met psychiatrist Chris Ivany (the other author of this book), then an Army major and chief of the Department of Behavioral Health at Evans Army Community Hospital, Fort Carson's medical facility. Two days earlier, Chris had received an unusual call from the office of the vice chief of staff of the Army, the four-star general supporting JK's team. Majors rarely get direct calls from offices so high up in the chain of command. Dr. Quinkert let him know that a small team from MIT would be visiting at the direction of General Chiarelli. Chris could not imagine what MIT had to do with the Army or behavioral health care, but he quickly rearranged his calendar to accommodate the request of the Army's second-most powerful officer.

Chris and his team at Fort Carson spent several days showing their visitors from Cambridge how mental health care was delivered at the Mountain Post. The Fort Carson team highlighted Embedded Behavioral Health (EBH), a model of care they had recently developed to provide outpatient mental health care to soldiers within walking distance of their workplaces.

Observing EBH at Fort Carson was a revelation to the MIT team. They saw the power of the working relationships that had developed between the EBH providers and the command teams. They witnessed a mental health care team in Iraq conducting a conference call with the EBH team at Fort Carson to discuss the care they were providing to a soldier who would soon be returning home and into the EBH team's care. The close coordination between providers employed by the hospital and those working as part of combat units in Iraq, even while the unit was deployed, was starkly different from what they had observed at other Army hospitals. The quantitative data analyzed by the MIT team reinforced the observation that Fort Carson was different from other locations. Patients got appointments more frequently, commanders observed that their soldiers were getting the care that they needed, and fewer needed to be placed in inpatient psychiatric wards. In a few short days, it became clear that Embedded Behavioral Health was a genuine improvement and would similarly benefit soldiers on other Army posts, but no system existed to take a best practice from one place and replicate it elsewhere.

Although it had not yet been put into practice, Army medical leaders were taking preliminary steps to create a system of mental health care built around best practices the MIT team envisioned. On March 1, 2011, Lieutenant General Eric Schoomaker, the Army surgeon general at the time, testified to the Senate Appropriations Committee about the Army's new Comprehensive Behavioral Health System of Care (CBHSOC), which was its campaign to create an integrated, coordinated, and synchronized behavioral health service delivery system.[5]

After the first round of site visits, JK and his graduate students consolidated their initial findings and the team captured stories of the challenges soldiers and families faced in navigating a constantly changing system of care. The MIT team also reported the differences between locations in terms of volume and intensity of mental health care use. One location continued to stand out: Fort Carson. It was the only place where leaders, soldiers, and others expressed to the team confidence in their mental health care system.

General Chiarelli was set to retire in early 2012, and he asked for an update on where we were on the project before that. On January 17, 2012, the MIT team reported to him our findings: mental health care on a lot of Army posts had been reduced to doing psychiatric triage rather than actually improving soldier health. When he asked whether things were working well anywhere, the team pointed to Fort Carson and the positive impact Embedded Behavioral Health was having. He asked us to share our findings with a larger group a few days later.

The next Saturday, General Chiarelli gathered several senior leaders at the Pentagon. The MIT team wasn't aware that he had also arranged for the meeting to include a videoconference with the commanding general on every Army post across the world. After the MIT team shared its findings and recommendation to replicate EBH, General Chiarelli gave his full-throated endorsement and directed Lieutenant General Horoho, the new Army surgeon general, to rearrange her hospital's outpatient mental health care clinics to support the EBH model. The surgeon general's staff reassigned Chris Ivany from Fort Carson to its headquarters in Falls Church, Virginia, to work as part of the burgeoning mental health leadership team and spearhead EBH implementation. General Chiarelli's meeting also opened the doors for the MIT team to make visits to many other Army posts to continue to observe and learn.

In 2013, the surgeon general selected Chris to serve as the chief of the Behavioral Health Division and lead the team charged with improving mental health services throughout the Army. The partnership between JK and Chris continued over the next three years and included twenty-seven field visits to nineteen Army locations between 2012 and 2015.

Through open conversations that only outsiders could have, JK and his team won the trust of countless people involved in Army behavioral health care who frequently disclosed how things were really working at the local level. Chris and his team incorporated that perspective to identify and solve problems they may not have found otherwise. This insider-outsider relationship enabled JK to serve as a neutral observer of the change effort and understand the Army culture well enough to make relevant recommendations.

This book tells the story of the Army's transformation of that disparate collection of poorly standardized and largely disconnected clinical microsystems into a well-defined mental health care system with patient-centered, recovery-oriented care as its foundation, which uses real-time knowledge to improve patient outcomes, measure performance, and reward high-value care. It is a step-by-step explication of *how* this was accomplished that offers profound lessons about the provision of behavioral health services and can help guide other mental health care systems across the country as well to transform into *learning* mental health care systems.

Today, the Army has overcome what was once a kind of "organized anarchy" to achieve a standardized system of care—an important step toward ensuring a consistent care experience irrespective of care location. It also establishes care ownership, a necessary prerequisite for patient-centered care. The Army's transformed system of care provides transparency of patient flows, visibility to care delivered, and conformance to workload standards. The Army is building the capability to go beyond proxy measures to use patient-reported outcomes to answer whether beneficiaries are actually getting better. The foundations of a *learning health care system* that can measure performance and improve quality of care have taken root.

Who This Book Is For

We've written this book for health systems leaders and policy makers looking to make the major changes to their health care systems necessary for them to become *learning* health care systems. The profound desire to address the mental health crises that have manifested in soldiers and their families over the last twenty years created an opportunity to change the Army's mental health system more extensively and more rapidly than in any other period of history. This book tells the story of the Army's transformation of that disparate collection of poorly standardized and largely disconnected clinics into a well-defined mental health care system with patient-centered, recovery-oriented care as its foundation, using real-time knowledge to improve patient outcomes, measure performance, and reward high-value care. This book is a step-by-step explication of *how* this was accomplished. The Army's experience offers profound lessons about the provision of behavioral health services and can help guide mental health care systems across the country in their own transformations into *learning* mental health care systems.

This book codifies what did and did not work in the Army's transformation efforts. The framework we develop here is based on the Army's experience, but we believe the lessons are applicable to all health systems—civilian systems, other public health systems such as the Veterans Affairs system, and the other branches of the military.

The Army is a useful case example because it is an integrated care delivery system in which policy guidance and management are centralized. We do not suggest that health systems try to replicate the Army's behavioral health system of care exactly, but rather take the core ideas and use them to build their own learning mental health care systems. These ideas include gaining an accurate, empirically supported understanding of the current state of their mental health care system, including the flow of patients across levels of care; proactively redesigning the system of care around patient needs to create a consistent, culturally competent patient experience of care; focusing on reducing and ultimately eliminating the stigma of using mental health care services; systematically collecting and using patient-reported outcomes as the foundation for the learning health care system; and implementing a practice management system that provides leaders with a clear understanding of the actual clinical care provided.

In understanding the Army's journey, we believe leaders and policy makers can guide their own health systems to make the major changes necessary for building learning health care systems.

As we completed this book, health systems around the world were grappling not just with treating patients with Covid-19, but also with the pandemic's impact on the mental health of patients, clinical care teams, and the public writ large. It is even more important now to treat mental health care and medical care within a unified health system. Unfortunately, civilian health care systems are still dealing with the aftereffects of deinstitutionalization, when much of mental health care shifted away from the hospitals and into independent community-based clinics and practices.[6] This created a fissure between medical and mental health care that was widened even further by funding approaches, such as mental health carve-outs, established to manage the growing costs of mental health care. Efforts to restore parity, such as the Mental Health Parity and Addiction Equity Act of 2008, increased access to mental health care services and accelerated the adoption of patient-centric care models such collaborative care models that provide behavioral health care in primary care settings.[7] Unfortunately, these successes have generally been limited to single initiatives and have not achieved the redesign of the entire system that is required to fix the country's profound mental health care challenges.

In contrast, the Army *did* redesign its entire mental health care system. We describe the transformation from a provider-centric, stovepiped system with unchecked variation between its clinics to a patient-centered, integrated, and cohesive system of care based on patient-reported outcome data. The book organizes the Army's lessons learned into a framework leaders can use to build mental health care systems that learn and improve over time. Beginning with systematically understanding the behavioral health care needs of the health systems' beneficiaries, health systems can establish a structure of empowered leaders to redesign and reorganize its clinics around the needs of patients. We lay out the core management components that every health system needs to manage its mental health care practice effectively to enable learning across all levels of the health system, including the measurement of clinical outcomes, a performance management system that connects health system objectives to actual clinical care, a roadmap for selecting and growing leaders, and an implementation framework for translating learning across the health system into practice.

In the midst of responding to Covid-19, the military is also transforming its health system. It is establishing a single organization, the Defense Health Agency (DHA), to manage the hospitals previously run independently by the Army, Navy, and Air Force. This agency now has the mandate to do for the Department of Defense what Chris and team did for the Army: identify best practices, standardize them across the enterprise, and improve them based on how patients say they perform. As with any large bureaucracy, the risk is to standardize to the least common denominator, which has the potential of undermining the progress the Army has made. The DHA has taken positive steps toward preserving core principles that enabled the Army to build a learning mental health system. But much more work, and risk, lies ahead.

This book provides a framework that military health system policy makers and leaders in any health system can use to guide their efforts to build a learning mental health system.

Chapter 1

ORGANIZED ANARCHY IN ARMY MENTAL HEALTH CARE

While serving as the chief of the Department of Behavioral Health at the hospital at Fort Carson, Colorado, Chris received a call from the chief of one of the behavioral health clinics on the post. She pleasantly asked Chris to drive the mile or so over to see something unusual that had just arrived in her clinic. She preferred not to describe it over the phone. Slightly annoyed at the disruption to his morning schedule, Chris arrived a few minutes later. Sitting on the desk in the office of one of the psychologists was a large rock, about ten pounds, nearly a foot around and painted bright pink. Not understanding what he was looking at, Chris asked the psychologist for an explanation.

She said that a private first class (a very junior soldier who has been in the Army less than two years) had lugged the curious object with him to an appointment with her earlier this morning. Confused, she asked him why he had the conspicuous object. He calmly stated that his first sergeant (a noncommissioned officer serving in an important leadership role) had made a new rule in his company (a small Army unit of about one hundred soldiers).

"What's the new rule?" the psychologist inquired.

Matter-of-factly, the soldier explained that anyone in his company who is unable to train with the unit, or who has a pending medical discharge for a mental health condition, is required to carry a large pink rock everywhere he or she goes.

The year is 2010.

Shocked, Chris wondered, "Why was this first sergeant, an experienced leader, intentionally embarrassing his soldiers and discouraging them from taking advantage of mental health care the Army offered?" If we take a step back and consider the situation from the first sergeant's perspective, we may be able to see the full scope of the problem.

The first sergeant, like all Army leaders in charge of combat units, was under incredible pressure to get his company ready for its next deployment, now only six months away. He had felt the pain of losing soldiers in combat in the past, and this time he was determined to bring all of his soldiers home alive. That meant everyone had to be fully trained and ready.

But mental health problems kept cropping up, often in his best soldiers. Some appeared depressed, angry, and less interested in the mission. They'd miss critical training events to go to appointments at the Army hospital. Sometimes, they'd come back with paperwork that said they couldn't be around weapons for the next month or two—no small thing in an infantry unit. And most of them didn't seem to be getting any better anyway—at least not as the first sergeant saw it.

At one point, he had fifteen of his soldiers in treatment. He would call the hospital to track down the twelve different behavioral health providers (psychiatrists, psychologists, clinical social workers, or nurse practitioners) treating those soldiers, trying to find out which of them were not going to be able to deploy with the rest of the company when the time came. When he left voice mails, only a few of the providers called him back. When he did reach someone, he got little more than a cryptic "lecture" about the difficulty of predicting how mental health conditions respond to treatment—meaning no answer to his question. Frustrated, confused, and angry, he decided to take matters into his own hands and discourage any more of his soldiers from getting tangled up in what seemed to him the morass that was Army behavioral health care.

Why would the first sergeant decide to make an already difficult situation for soldiers worse by attaching even more stigma to their conditions? Because the Army had failed to offer a system that helped him to take care of his soldiers and address his primary concern of getting his company ready for their next deployment.

This *real* story reveals a few of the numerous problems that plagued the Army's early attempts to combat the rising tide of mental illness brought on by the wars in Iraq and Afghanistan. Overcoming these and many others would take a near total transformation of the clinical system that organized, delivered, and monitored the care.

Understanding Learning Health Systems

In 2013, the National Academy of Medicine published a consensus report that articulated the vision for a learning health system as one "in which science, informatics, incentives, and culture are aligned for continuous improvement and innovation, with best practices seamlessly embedded in the care process, patients and families active participants in all elements, and new knowledge captured as an integral by-product of the care experience."[1] This report consolidated the findings from a series of eleven learning health systems publications, beginning with the proceedings of the first workshop in 2007 that described the need for building a learning health system and including ten subsequent volumes addressing specific components of the learning health system model, ranging from evidence generation to leadership.[2] Figure 1.1 shows a schematic of a learning health system. With this series, the National Academies Press continues to capture insights from the nation's leading experts on the components of building learning health systems (LHS).[3]

LHS represent a fundamental shift in the design of health systems in general and mental health systems in particular, because of the historical separation between mental health care and other medical care, the disciplinary fragmentation that exists within mental health care, and the stigma associated with having a mental health condition.[4]

Learning health systems share several attributes relevant for our discussion here. They have systems of care designed around the needs and perspectives of patients and the community served. Clinicians are trained to be respectful of those

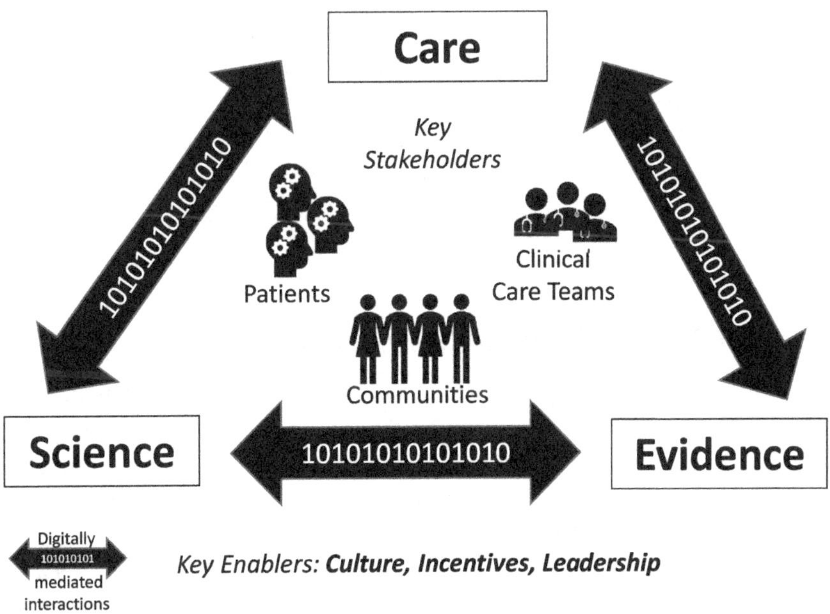

FIGURE 1.1. Learning health system. Adapted from Institute of Medicine, *Best Care at Lower Cost.*

needs and perspectives. LHS have digital infrastructures to capture the patient experience of care reliably. They are transparent in their use of data to improve the care experience, care quality, and care outcomes. They improve clinical decision making by providing clinicians with the best evidence available. They utilize incentives designed to promote high-value care. And finally, LHS leaders promote a culture of learning.

In 2010, the Army's mental health care system was not designed with those attributes in mind. Each Army hospital had its own unique mental health care system that had evolved based on local needs and local provider interests. Commanders, one of the most important stakeholders, felt the mental health system was not taking care of their soldiers. Many clinicians were not trained to understand the Army culture, making it difficult for them to understand soldiers and provide culturally competent care.

The Army's digital infrastructure was long in the tooth, and it was not designed to support mental health care. The administrative data did not map effectively to the actual clinical care provided to soldiers and family members. Known delays in the analysis and reporting of even the high-level administrative data meant that Army hospitals could not use that data to understand and address deficiencies in the patient experience or care quality.

Like most mental health systems, the Army's had no systematic means of assessing whether the care provided was actually making patients better. Given that the Army did not have an automated process for systematically collecting patient reported outcomes, it was left to individual providers to manually collect, analyze, and incorporate data into their clinical decision making. The Army did not provide to Army hospitals incentives that were specifically focused on improving mental health outcomes; rather, it focused on process measures related to enhancing access for soldiers returning from an overseas combat tour.

From Stable Demand to Organized Anarchy

A learning health system cannot be built if there is no defined system of care. When the MIT research team initially tried to answer the simple question about how the Army organized and delivered mental health care, the team was surprised to learn that even the Army had no clear understanding for its thirty-three military treatment facilities. There was a high-level definition of the care being provided in the *direct care system* (care delivered in Army hospitals) or as *purchased care*—care sourced from civilian health care systems near an Army post, where service members could use their TRICARE insurance.

Prior to 2006, mental health care in the Army was delivered at Army hospitals in separate departments: psychiatry, psychology, and social work. This traditional organizational structure made it easier to recruit providers because the departments corresponded to national academic training programs, professional societies, licensure boards, and certification agencies with which these providers dealt outside the military. The Army could easily determine what providers could and could not do, and it could authorize them to provide care within their scope of practice. A soldier or family member would access services within a given department as needed. For complex cases requiring that a soldier or family member be seen in multiple departments, case coordination would often be left to those individual care providers.

Even though there was some variation in care offerings across the different hospitals, demand grew slowly from 4.44 percent of *all active-duty soldiers* using mental health care services in 2003 to 6.46 percent in 2006.[5] The department-based design had been able to meet the needs of those soldiers and their families.

Then things began to change rapidly. The ongoing wars in Afghanistan and Iraq placed significantly more demands on the Army. By 2011, soldiers had spent more than 1.5 million troop-years in a combat setting, a 28 percent increase from 2007. About 73 percent of active and reserve soldiers and National Guard members had deployed to Iraq and Afghanistan, and most were on their second, third, or fourth year of cumulative deployed duty.[6] The period 2007 to 2010 saw the sharpest growth in the use of mental health services. Outpatient visits nearly doubled as the percentage of active-duty soldiers using mental health care services spiked from 7.7 to 12.4 percent. Inpatient admissions also shot upward, from 16,794 to 23,680.[7]

At the same time, a number of external and internal reports about the situation created a real sense of urgency to increase access to mental health care services. The Dole-Shalala Commission, convened in response to a series of articles in the *Washington Post* that documented poor conditions, neglect, and bureaucratic hurdles faced by outpatients at Walter Reed Army Medical Center, released a report "proving to the American public that the Walter Reed fiasco [was] just the tip of the iceberg."[8] The RAND Corporation released a report as part of its Invisible Wounds of War Project that found evidence to suggest that "the psychological toll" of deployments to Afghanistan and Iraq "may be disproportionately high compared with the physical injuries of combat."[9] Internal findings by the Army's mental health assessment teams and the DoD Task Force on Mental Health also stoked the calls for change.[10]

In 2007, when the US Congress added more than $200 million annually for Army hospitals to improve access to mental health care, there was very little direction from the Army surgeon general to Army hospitals on how to spend those funds. Army hospitals rapidly created dozens of new programs, and by 2010 there were more than sixty unique clinical programs across the Army.[11] Independent of the Army's own efforts, a team of MIT students tried to figure out what all the programs actually did.[12] They had a list of program names and locations, but nothing more. Six graduate students working half-time every day for three months looked for information on the Web, found phone numbers, and then called the hospitals and the nonclinical agencies on Army posts, trying to get some explanation of what the programs did. We identified some programs that were labeled "mental health care" that actually focused on nonclinical supportive activities such as yoga and aromatherapy. What had once been a stable system design—even if services were not what they needed to be—had become *organized anarchy*.[13]

A System Design That Did Not Promote Care Seeking

When the MIT team completed its first round of visits to six Army bases, it became abundantly clear that each base had a unique mental health care system.[14] These systems were not patient-centric, and most of the clinical care was still delivered at the base hospital. Soldiers and family members had to navigate across multiple programs in multiple departments to find the right care.

At one Army post, the MIT team discovered four different entry points into the mental health care system: a soldier could make an appointment with the behavioral health department; she could receive mental health services in the substance abuse clinic or from her unit behavioral health providers; or she could be referred to a civilian health care system near the post. At another post, all soldiers could enter the mental health care system only through a centralized triage clinic. Even after they were triaged to the appropriate mental health clinic, they were not permitted to receive mental health care services in the substance use clinic or from their unit behavioral health providers. There was no shared understanding across all the key gatekeepers—chaplains, commanders, family members, and other medical providers—about where soldiers would receive care after that first visit.

The sheer variation in how soldiers and family members accessed care from one post to the next was really a problem. More than a third of the Army population moves every year, meaning soldiers and their families, had to discover new ways to get care again and again. The MIT team analyzed administrative data and found that almost half the soldiers who were in treatment before a move did not follow up on that treatment after moving to another post. It was impossible to be sure, but the team suspected that was due to the differences in each hospital's behavioral health care programs.

The real anarchy, though—the kind we immediately realized had a terribly negative impact on soldiers seeking care—was in the confusion over where to get care, and how the available care from one post to another was so inconsistent. This confusion even extended to how programs and services were named.

At Fort Hood, Texas, for example, the Army built a "Resilience and Restoration Center" with four clinics that provided the full spectrum of services from routine care to urgent care, to a specialized PTSD treatment program.[15] But a soldier moving from Fort Hood to Fort Bliss, also in Texas, would find at the latter a Restoration and Resilience Center, with the terms confusingly reversed, that provided *only* PTSD treatment.[16] In other words, soldiers and family members who successfully overcame the stigma associated with seeking mental health care in the Army couldn't even find a consistent pathway to access care. The system was not designed to do that.

Growing Disconnect between Providers and Commanders

In 2010, too many soldiers could not perform their duties because of mental illness and, as a result, weren't able to train with their units or deploy with them to Iraq or Afghanistan. There was continual wrangling between military leaders and care providers, pulling soldiers in different directions. Leaders felt urgency to deploy at full strength to fight the wars in Iraq and Afghanistan; mental health care providers felt soldiers were not getting the time and support needed to recover. Soldiers were stuck in the middle.

Very few mental health providers regularly talked with unit leaders such as the first sergeant in the pink rock story to provide advice or to answer questions about how to manage and support soldiers with mental health issues. On many large posts, soldiers waited more than four weeks for an initial appointment. Rising suicide rates increased the pressure on military leaders, care providers, and others who increasingly pointed fingers of blame at one another—failing to recognize that the real problem was the Army mental health *system* itself. In this environment, is it any wonder that individual providers, clinic chiefs, hospital commanders, and even first sergeants were trying to come up with their own solutions, including ones that featured brightly colored rocks?

Soldiers and family members expect behavioral health care to meet their social, cultural, and linguistic needs—in other words, they expect care to be delivered in a culturally competent manner. The onus of achieving this objective is not only on the care system, but also on individual care providers. As challenging as achieving cultural competence in health care is generally, it may be even more difficult when providers are not accustomed to the Army's unique context.

The Army ideal is to provide mental health services in a manner that reflects the diverse values, beliefs, and behaviors of soldiers and their families. This is especially difficult because the mix of providers in the direct care system has changed dramatically from largely uniformed personnel to more than three-fourths civilian providers. Many of these care providers have no previous experience either in the military or working with a military population.

This creates challenges. For instance, even though English is the Army's operational language, soldiers and their families use slang that for nonmilitary people can seem like a completely different language. Providers must become reasonably proficient in "Army-speak." But how many civilians, for instance, know that to "go ruck" means to go on a training exercise and walk with full equipment? It's a word that shows up in Army-speak every day. Then there is all the terminology the Army uses that may not exist in the civilian world or may have completely different meanings, such as "profile," which is actually a detailed description of duty limitations—that is, what a soldier can and cannot do from an operational sense; the closest, but still not very close, equivalent might be the note a worker brings to the boss from his doctor.[17]

Understanding the medical conditions that may limit the ability of soldiers to deploy into combat is another cultural competency challenge.[18] For instance, changing the dose of an antidepressant medication to address an annoying side effect, such as an upset stomach, is routine in the civilian world. But that same change would render a soldier ineligible to go to Iraq or Afghanistan with her/his unit because the Army requires a soldier to be stable for at least three months on a psychiatric medicine before going to a combat zone. Circumstances such as these can be sources of considerable friction for the soldier and the unit that was counting on the soldier as an integral part of the team.

The military exception to the Health Insurance Portability and Accountability Act (HIPAA) also adds some complexity to behavioral health care in the Army. In the civilian setting, the patient's employer is entitled to little or no information about the patient's health status. In the military, because other soldiers' well-being often depends on the soldier-patient's ability to perform his or her job, health care providers are required to let commanders know if the patient cannot do so.[19] Some providers did not have a clear understanding of military applications of HIPAA and were unwilling to share information with commanders despite the exception. The lack of communication left many commanders uneasy about soldiers dealing with mental health problems and contributed to the stigma of seeking care.

One of the core challenges before implementation was the adversarial relationship between command teams and behavioral health care providers that was continually fueled by perceived differences in goals and interests.[20] The Army's goal of readiness was interpreted by commanders as *readiness to deploy* and by providers as *function restoration*. Commanders saw mental health as a medical problem and the hospitals as not servicing their soldiers appropriately. They worried that use of mental health services was taking away from their fighting force, and that mental health providers were reluctant to share information regarding the health and recovery of the soldier receiving services. Providers saw commanders as uncaring, and in some cases as stigmatizing soldiers who used behavioral health care services. Commanders used mental status evaluations as a means of extracting information from providers, while providers used formal documentation to create a paper trail that forced commanders to take explicit ownership of the decision to deploy a soldier the provider felt should remain behind.

Redesigning Care around Needs of Soldiers, Providers, and Commanders

A series of reports pointing to rising suicide rates, along with these other problems, led the Army to recognize an urgent need to create consistent patient experiences.[21] Whether a soldier received care at Fort Polk, Louisiana, or Camp Red Cloud, Korea, the Army set out to develop a standard system of care that would identify the ideal pathways that a soldier could use to seek mental health care, the flow across the different clinics that would form the system of care, and the staffing and management of those different clinics.

By 2010, clinics were being supported using core DoD health care funding, new funds from Congress allocated specifically for mental health, supplemental funds for fighting the wars in Iraq and Afghanistan, research funds, and even foundation funding for special programs such as the National Intrepid Center of Excellence.[22] The Army, replicating part of what our graduate students had done, also set out to identify the different programs and clinics involved through a painstaking process that required hospital leaders to report to headquarters what they had in their local system of care and identify the funds that supported those programs.

Increased funding alone, though, was not going to fix the problem. The Army needed to reorganize how it provided care. So, fourteen working groups that brought together subject matter experts from across the Army began to meet to define the requirements for a standard patient-centric system of care.[23] The groups found consensus on the key components of the system such as family care, soldier

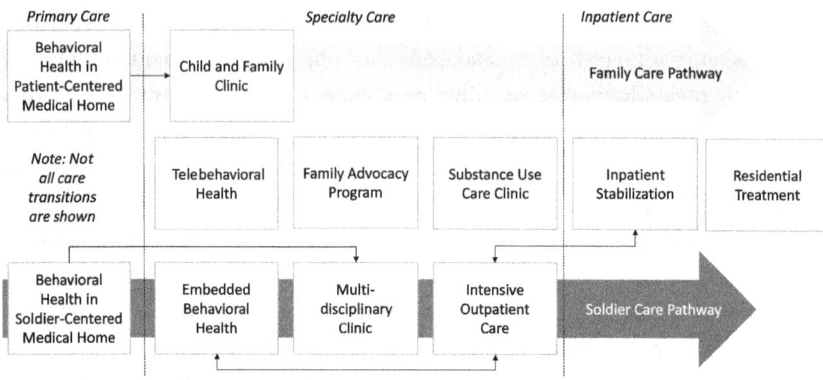

FIGURE 1.2. Design of the Army behavioral health system of care in 2017

care, and telebehavioral health. These working groups also focused on key enabling processes, such as outcome measurement, incentives, and governance, and built the foundation that led to critically needed changes in policy and organizing. Figure 1.2 shows the result: a design for a reorganized Army Behavioral Health System of Care (BHSOC).

For the first time, the Army had clearly defined core clinical microsystems and patient care pathways between them.[24] Each clinical microsystem would be expected to conform to Army-wide standards for staffing and the population of beneficiaries served (the "catchment area"). The design of the BHSOC prioritized *soldier* care by clearly defining separate care pathways for soldiers and other beneficiaries. The telebehavioral system in particular was a recognition that the capacity to provide care, especially in the remote areas where Army posts are usually located, simply did not correspond to demand. Beyond bridging that gap in the short term, the technology was important both in terms of long-term, sustainable capacity *expansion* and to provide surge capacity when needed in locations with significant provider shortages.

The BHSOC standardized design became the template for all Army hospitals, but it did not require every hospital to implement every component of the system. For instance, because there is insufficient demand to warrant providing acute inpatient care within the *direct care* system on every post, these services are sourced from the *purchased care* network at those locations. Nor is the BHSOC set in stone. Developing new programs is not ruled out; rather, the new design enables hospitals to be more deliberate about understanding population needs and developing justifications for new programs.

After all the financial investments by the Army and Congress and the intensive design efforts by the Army's Behavioral Health leadership at the system level, key questions remained unanswered: Are soldiers and their families willing to seek mental health care? Does the system have the right data and tools to support data-driven decision making by clinicians and administrators? Does the care provided improve health outcomes for soldiers and their families?

The Army had taken a big step forward with the standardized design. But a design to address a problem is only as good as its implementation.

Stigma Negatively Affected Use of Mental Health Care

When the external study team asked soldiers whether they were willing to seek mental health care, there was a range of responses—most of them essentially "no."

"Nah," one said. "I tried, but the clinic is so backed up that they can't see me for another six weeks."

"Why bother?" said another. "Mental health care doesn't work."

"No way I'm going," said a third, "because it will end my career."

These responses revealed the lived reality of soldiers in 2010. Clinics were severely overextended and soldiers often had to wait more than six weeks between outpatient visits—big delays driven partly by the lack of sufficient capacity to meet the growing need for services and partly by poorly designed organizational metrics. The Army realized it had to do *something*, so it mandated that soldiers returning from combat zones were to be provided "enhanced access to care," meaning they had to be seen within seven days of requesting an appointment.[25] Some hospitals responded by setting up triage clinics so they could meet the letter of this "law," and they succeeded in making sure that everyone was seen for their first visit within those seven days. The Army, however, had made no additional stipulation regarding follow-up other than the standard follow-up of twenty-eight days. There was just too much demand to meet even that!

All in all, this exacerbated an already bad situation. Soldiers found themselves having to tell their story multiple times to multiple providers before establishing a sustained care relationship. It was not a system that got the soldier into the right care at the right time—further contributing to the underlying narrative that Army mental health care did not work.

Specialist Williams returned from his second tour of duty in Afghanistan needing mental health services. First, he had to go to the triage clinic at his stateside installation, where a provider conducted a fifteen-minute assessment to determine whether he was at immediate risk to harm himself or others. That provider concluded that Specialist Williams was not a risk, and referred him to a different clinic on post where he went through a longer assessment process. It wasn't lost on

Specialist Williams that this second appointment seemed to be just like starting over; he was covering a lot of the same ground, with many of the questions exactly the same as what he'd been asked in the first assessment—even though the Army had an electronic medical record on him that should have included the results of the initial assessment.

Soldiers like Specialist Williams, in 2010, would have to go through six visits on average before moving from the "assessment" phase to an actual psychiatric diagnostic interview. No wonder soldiers and leaders were complaining.

To complicate things, many soldiers worried that even using mental health care services would have a negative impact on their career. Specialist Williams's decision to go to the triage clinic in the first case was made with great trepidation. Like everyone else in his unit, he knew that soldiers who used inpatient mental health care services were very likely to be discharged from the Army within a year.[26] Soldiers also did not want to be seen as weak by their peers and their leaders, and they genuinely feared that mental health providers were sharing all the information from therapy sessions with the soldier's leadership team—even though very few providers in 2010 were consistently engaging with commanders.

These challenges to getting soldiers to the point where they were even *willing* to seek care were playing out within the larger context of stigma—an issue the Army had to address head-on. The Army made a significant investment in a stigma-reduction campaign in an effort to shift the culture from "avoiding care" to "care seeking," and in 2010 it worked with the DoD to revise Standard Form 86 to exclude explicitly seeking mental health services either for a family issue or for adjustments from service in a combat environment as potential barriers for obtaining a security clearance.[27]

Some soldiers were also wary of seeking mental health care due to the perception that doing so could lead to an administrative separation, which is a nonmedical process through which some soldiers are discharged from the Army, often with limited benefits. Soldiers can be administratively separated for many reasons, including misconduct or the inability to maintain their weight within the required standard. In other cases, soldiers are administratively separated when a lifelong behavioral health condition, such as personality disorder, creates occupational problems during active duty, or when soldiers cannot do their job due to a nondisabling condition, such as an adjustment disorder due to an inability to adapt to life in the military. There were real concerns that Army commanders were inappropriately using administrative separations to quickly discharge soldiers with serious mental health problems, such as depression and PTSD, rather than going through the long and onerous disability evaluation and medical retirement process.

Perhaps the most contentious scenario is when a soldier with a mental health condition commits one or more acts of misconduct, and the commander responds by pursuing an administrative separation—even though the Army has a process by which it is supposed to consider carefully the soldier's mental health condition as a mitigating factor for the alleged misconduct. The situation is especially charged if the commander seeks an adverse characterization, such as an "Other Than Honorable" discharge, which can have lifelong ramifications.[28] In response, the Army refined its policies on the role of behavioral health providers in administrative separations and strengthened oversight of the medical aspect of the process.[29]

New Tools Needed to Support Administrative Decision Making

The planning tools the Army used before implementing the standard system of care estimated required capacity based on the known demand for care and local leadership guesstimates of expected demand in subsequent years. There was no way to account systematically for the increase in demand that was becoming the norm from soldiers immediately on their return from Iraq or Afghanistan. Behavioral health clinics became backlogged, and because they had to prioritize care for the sickest patients, delays for other patients further increased the use of emergency department care and ultimately led to more inpatient admissions (as figure 1.3 shows).

After the new system of care was specified in 2010, it took another three years before the Army was ready to mandate and assess implementation. In the intervening period, 2011 to 2013, use of outpatient mental health services continued to grow, albeit at a slower rate, from 2.9 to more than 3.3 million visits. Inpatient admissions for mental health reasons actually dropped from 26,281 to 25,597.

To create the capacity for mental health care that would allow for implementing the BHSOC, the Army knew it would have to transform the discipline-based organization into one that used multidisciplinary care teams within the standardized clinics. Doing so would require developing new workload standards to reflect the full spectrum of work performed: clinical work taking care of soldiers and their families *and* nonclinical activities such as consulting with commanders and preparing occupational or "duty" evaluations, which assess the impact of the soldier's mental health condition on their ability to perform their job in the Army.[30] And it would mean establishing both new productivity requirements for providers *and* new ways to measure productivity. Typically, only the clinical workload

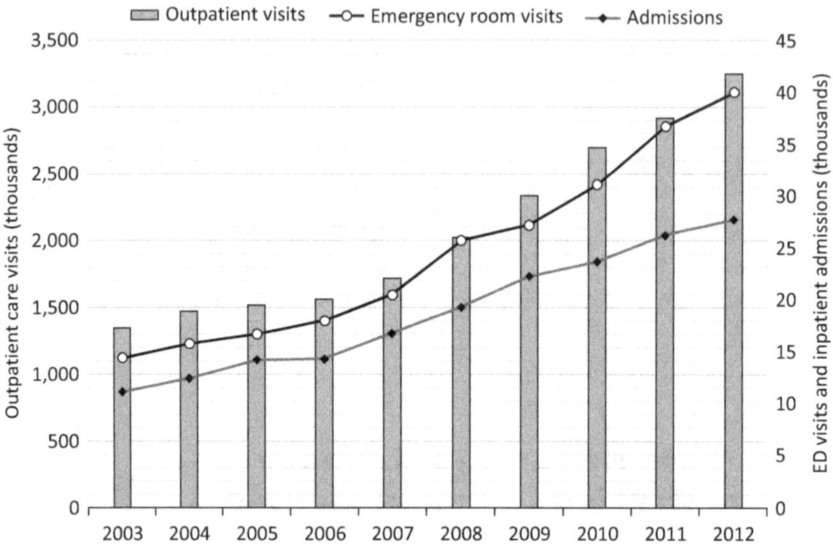

FIGURE 1.3. Consistent increase in utilization of mental health care over time

is measured, because it is prioritized, but the Army would need to measure all the other nonclinical, but nevertheless essential, work activities in which providers would be involved, such as education and command consultation. All this would require training providers and leaders on the new productivity standards, but also working with administrators and coders to ensure the measuring was accurate and captured in human resource systems.

The shift from design to implementation also required radical changes in how the Army assessed the performance of its mental health care. The Army created productivity assessment tools that integrated data from human resource management systems and administrative data systems to analyze and compare provider-level, clinic-level, and hospital-level performance against minimum expected standards of clinical care delivery.

The Army also needed to address how money was being spent at the local level. Some hospitals had begun to use the new funding provided by Congress (intended to create more clinical services to address soldiers' behavioral health problems) to pay instead for their existing behavioral health clinics. The hospitals then shifted the old behavioral health funds to other higher revenue-generating projects, such as improving surgical services. To change this, the Army centralized more decision-making authority on spending, taking away some of the discretionary power of the hospital leaders. These new constraints on hospitals were accompanied by education on the need to create a standard system of care that expanded access and improved quality.

Until 2014, Army leaders also had limited ability to monitor and improve systematically the patient experience of care (including quality and satisfaction), because the administrative data collected were incomplete, complex, and disorganized. Workflow accounting codes had evolved in an ad hoc manner from one hospital to the next, resulting in an unwieldy tangle of ninety-four inconsistently used codes to measure performance across dozens of different clinical programs. The Army revised its accounting codes to link each of the emerging standard system-wide clinical programs with a single standardized code, irrespective of geographic location. For the first time, the Army could directly compare the performance of a clinic in Honolulu, Hawaii, to one in Killeen, Texas.

Based on the improved administrative data, the Army also developed a performance management system that included new incentives that would award additional funding to hospitals that succeeded in accelerating the transformation.

Need to Improve Clinical Decision Support to Improve Outcomes

The transformation into a learning health system is successful only when clinicians can incorporate the best available evidence into their practice and involve patients in shared decision making. The Army's electronic medical record was not designed to support mental health workflows, and clinicians had to rely on their own notes to capture details of a patient's recovery. Army clinicians were not consistently collecting patient-reported outcome data through standardized scales, or incorporating such data for treatment planning. Why? Because it was labor intensive to collect data from patients manually, analyze it during the patient visit, and then use the findings as part of treatment planning. Clinicians had different perspectives on the right set of assessment scales based on their own training, so even when clinicians collected outcome measures they were not always using the same assessment scales. The cost of paper-based psychological tests, and the lack of administrative staff to carry out the number crunching before the soldier or family member walked into the clinician's office, were additional factors cited in our interviews.

One provider elegantly framed the challenge in an interview we conducted. "It is not that I don't want to use a standardized instrument for depression. I was trained using the Beck's Depression Inventory, but I have to pay for the tests. The Patient Health Questionnaire is free, but I don't like it. Anyway, I ask all the questions when I'm talking to my patients, so I don't see why I need to do it twice."[31]

The Army had to create a digitally enabled workflow. This required developing a completely new system, the Behavioral Health Data Portal (BHDP), through which patient-reported outcomes data were collected systematically and consistently, evaluated, graphed, and presented to clinicians so they could use it as part of clinical decision making, as well as to engage patients during treatment planning.

When such data are collected consistently, the Army can clearly assess whether care provided to soldiers and family members is actually improving their health. It serves as the foundation for using practice data to generate additional evidence and guide research—a necessary starting point for any learning health system. The BHDP also became one of the key venues for the Army to incorporate new evidence into the practice. For example, it became easy to standardize the measurement instruments used by all Army clinicians.

Beyond Anarchy

The Army has transformed an organized anarchy into a learning mental health care system that delivers a consistent patient-centered care experience, irrespective of hospital location. This book chronicles that journey. It details the building blocks of a learning health system and discusses the broader implications of the Army experience for other health systems, including in the civilian world.

The Army has the advantage of being an integrated delivery system with centralized policy making and implementation assessment capabilities. Other health systems (both civilian and military) have to address the arm's-length relationships between mental health care providers and the larger health care system, and the associated policy implementation challenges. Still, the components of the Army's learning mental health care system can be readily replicated by other health systems.

The starting point for the transformation was developing and empowering groups of leaders to manage the change. That is the focus of chapter 2.

Chapter 2

A BRIEF AND INCOMPLETE HISTORY OF US ARMY MENTAL HEALTH CARE

Humans have understood something about the psychological impact of war for as long as war has been around. In *The Odyssey*, Homer vividly portrayed his view of the challenges men face when returning from combat through the story of Odysseus, culminating in his gory murders of left-at-home wife Penelope's would-be suitors. American military history includes descriptions of "soldier's heart" in soldiers suffering from combat stress as far back as the Civil War.[1] In fact, even accounting for cultural differences between generations and the differences in the wars themselves, clear connections can be drawn between modern-day PTSD and soldiers' mental health conditions in all major US conflicts.[2]

The history of the US military medical system's response, however, is much more complex.

Mental Health Care in Combat

An Army psychiatrist named Thomas Salmon, while serving on the staff of the surgeon general in 1917, developed the first systematic effort to combat US psychiatric casualties on the western front of World War I. He orchestrated an approach, adapted from British and French experience, to place psychiatrists in small clinics located as close to the front lines as possible. "Forward psychiatry," as it came to be known, intercepted soldiers suffering from shell shock and other psychological maladies immediately after the appearance of their symptoms got them removed from the trenches.

Salmon was aware of the long-standing and debilitating conditions in British soldiers who, suffering from similar symptoms, had been evacuated all the way to the rear or even back to Great Britain. Determined to help American soldiers avoid the same fate, his forward-placed clinics offered a soldier a chance to rest while retaining his critical social connections with other soldiers in his unit and avoiding the stigma of being too mentally ill to fight. Rejuvenated and supported by his peers, the soldier was frequently able to return to his duty stations on the front lines.[3]

Over the next century, Salmon's approach became the foundation of US military mental health care during combat. Each subsequent war added to what Salmon had begun.[4] By the time American forces stormed into Iraq and Afghanistan, US military mental health personnel were organized and well prepared to execute the modern version of Salmon's strategy. Large Army combat units, such as divisions and brigades, had mental health providers and specially trained medics assigned to them. Medical facilities called combat support hospitals or medical clinics had mental health providers on staff. Combat and operational stress control units, comprised of dozens of personnel, spread out across each theater to rapidly identify and treat soldiers who were suffering from combat stress—the modern-day successor to shell shock identified by Salmon nearly a century earlier.

Clear guidance, in the form of several Army regulations and manuals, spelled out the best method for delivering mental health services to soldiers in a combat theater. Those instructions contained the cumulative lessons learned from decades of trial and error. They were also published by the Department of Defense and the Army and distributed to medical personnel across the force, who incorporated them into official training programs. Even leaders of combat units were trained on combat stress control.[5] This high level of attention and resources produced a high degree of standardization in the practices employed by military mental health personnel when treating soldiers in theater. The Army had reasonably ensured that soldiers in combat could expect to receive the best-known care available for their psychiatric conditions.

Mental Health Care for Soldiers at Home

The relative success of Salmon's approach to mental health on the front lines in World War I helped establish the beginnings of mental health care for soldiers at their home stations. In the 1920s, the Army began to recognize psychiatric conditions as major challenges. Schizophrenia was the single leading disease cause for medical discharge. The suicide rate was more than fifty soldiers per hundred thousand per year (about twice as high as in the 2010s). Seven of the largest military medical facilities, such as Walter Reed General Hospital in Washington, D.C., and Tripler General Hospital in Hawaii established full-time inpatient and outpatient psychiatric wards and clinics.[6] By the end of the interwar period, mental health care had established a foothold within military medicine.

That foothold expanded in the latter part of World War II, based in part on the contributions of luminaries in the civilian psychiatric community who joined active duty during the war. One of them, William Menninger—a psychiatrist and member of a famed family of psychiatrists—served as a brigadier general and guided the Army to many key realizations. They included admitting that the Army had an inadequate number of mental health providers, recognizing the problems created by the lack of integration between mental health and other medical services, and acknowledging the importance of interdisciplinary care teams that included psychologists and clinical social.[7] Unfortunately, these same problems would plague the Army's approach to mental health care for decades to come.

The Vietnam War opened with an established cadre of psychiatrists leading a group of mental health outpatient clinics and inpatient wards around the world. In 1966, 274 psychiatrists served on active duty, about twice as many as in 2018.[8] They identified that mental health conditions frequently manifested as behavioral problems and drug and alcohol abuse, but they were only beginning to recognize the long-term psychological impact of trauma. The term "post-traumatic stress disorder" wouldn't find its way into the national lexicon until the American Psychiatric Association included it in the third edition of the *Diagnostic and Statistical Manual* in 1980.

In the 1970s, the Army had an extensive mental health infrastructure, and soldiers, especially draftees, served for a relatively brief period of time. As a result, the Army's mental health system at home proved to be up to the task of providing treatment for soldiers during the short time before they left active service. The problems caused by unrecognized mental illness created by service in Vietnam would be borne by the VA, well after soldiers had departed the Army.

The absence of prolonged wars between Vietnam and the US invasion of Afghanistan in the month after the September 11, 2001, terrorist attacks meant the Army's mental health system at home hadn't received a "stress test" in the decades preceding that war and the one in Iraq. And as the wars began, all seemed well.

Beginning in 2004, soldiers and their families began to show worrying signs associated with the stress from an increased "operational tempo," the Army's term for the frequency and duration of deployments (some lasting as long as fifteen months), which often included repeated exposure to combat-related trauma, but also includes the usual demands of Army life that involve regular moves and geographic separations between soldier and family.[9] Rates of depression, PTSD, anxiety disorders, and substance use disorders skyrocketed to levels never before

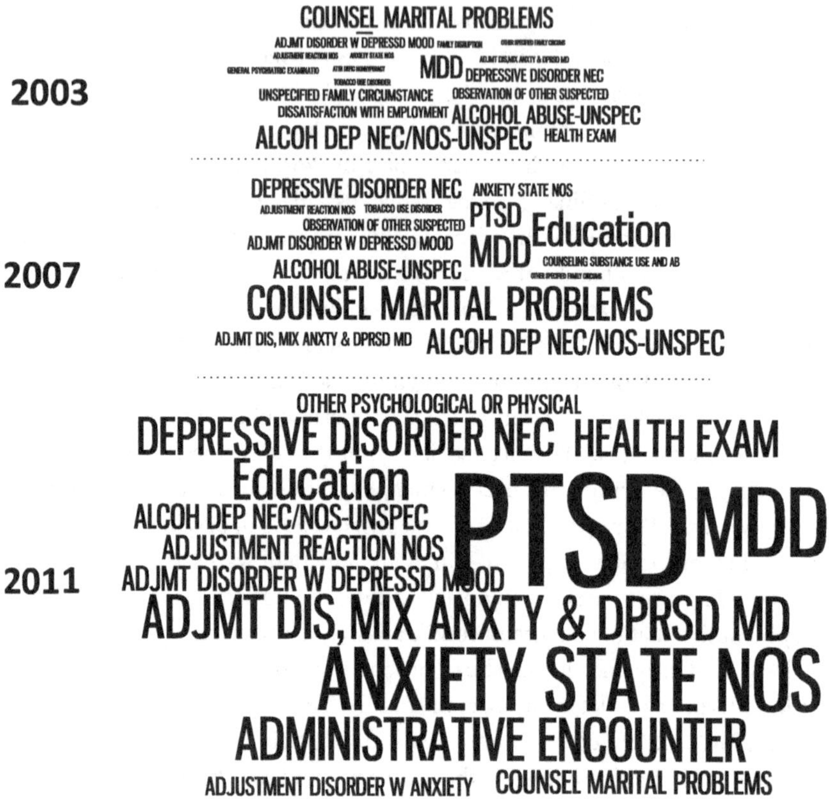

FIGURE 2.1. Changing nature of care in Army behavioral health

seen, creating a series of pressing issues for soldiers, their families, care providers, and unit leaders. It was a tremendous change in what Army mental health care providers needed to do for soldiers, as figure 2.1 shows.

Army Hospitals Struggle to Respond during the Global War on Terror

Imagine you live in a medium-size city somewhere in the United States, largely surrounded by small towns and mountains. On the news one day in early December, you hear the shocking story of an execution-style killing on a street in one of the quiet, middle-class neighborhoods of your city. A man delivering newspapers discovered a body on the sidewalk in a pool of blood, next to a picket fence decorated for Christmas. The victim had been shot twice in the head, at very close range.

A few nights later, a SWAT team surrounds a man at a local gas station and takes him into custody, charged with first-degree murder. Case closed? The man was with three others the night of the shooting, and on a hunch, investigators dig deeper. That digging implicates the group in a string of violent crimes in the surrounding area over the previous year.

It turns out that the previous summer, two of the men fired shots at a man who had run out of gas and was walking to a gas station; he was hit once, in the shoulder. Then they executed another man in a parking lot; that happened a week later, as the man begged for his life. A couple of months later, one of the men stabbed a nineteen-year-old nursing student six times; that happened after he had run her over with his vehicle. The detectives also figured out there had been a drive-by shooting; no one was hurt, but the lead investigator's gut told him there were plenty of incidents they didn't yet know about.

None of this is imaginary. If it seems familiar, you may have read an article about it in a newspaper or a very detailed story in *Rolling Stone* magazine, or seen coverage on television.[10] If it really hits home, you probably live in or near Colorado Springs, Colorado.

In addition to those small towns and mountains, there's an Army post nearby: Fort Carson. The man arrested for the execution-style murder in December had been recently court-martialed from the Army for stockpiling drugs in the barracks. He was with two other men that night, both of whom he had served with in the same unit in Iraq. One was a medic who had previously been arrested while on leave; the charge was beating his wife. The other was a private who had been diagnosed with PTSD and had, as another soldier put it, "started acting like King Kong."

The execution-style killing and the other incidents investigators uncovered were only a part of a larger problem.

In a series of highly publicized cases in Colorado Springs between 2005 and 2008, fourteen soldiers—twelve of whom had previously deployed to Iraq or Afghanistan—were charged with homicide, with attempted homicide, or as an accessory to homicide. In the aftermath, Army public health investigators seeking to understand what had contributed to the rash of violence found multiple converging factors, including high rates of exposure to combat related trauma, substance abuse, and histories of criminal behavior, even before the deployment. They also looked closely at how behavioral health problems may have played a part. Ten of the fourteen soldiers had a behavioral health condition, most commonly PTSD or depression.

In interviews by investigators after their arrests, the soldiers painted the picture of an overwhelmed Department of Behavioral Health, describing the care from the local Army hospital as "chaotic, sporadic, and uncaring." Of the nine soldiers confined at the time of the interviews, four stated they did not know how or where to get behavioral health help, and five felt they were not provided enough or the right type of care.[11]

In fact, at that time, the behavioral health clinics on Fort Carson had only 65 percent of the intended staffing level. Clinical teams tirelessly treated many more soldiers dealing with serious mental health problems than they were equipped to handle. The brigade to which most of the crime-committing soldiers belonged, for example, tripled its use of behavioral health care after returning from combat. Unable to manage the surge in demand for care, the hospital had resorted to referring soldiers en masse to civilian providers off the post and, in some cases, dispensing medications rather than providing much needed, but time-consuming, psychotherapy.[12]

Questions about the quality of the care was further called into question when a soldier with apparent psychotic symptoms, including delusions that he was an "alien dinosaur-like creature," was treated for a brief period by the behavioral health department, reportedly was declared "fit for duty," and then allegedly raped and killed a local teenager.[13]

Many other soldiers who may have benefitted from care were hesitant to seek it. Investigators also found high levels of stigma, or negative attitudes about mental health care and those receiving it, among soldiers on the post. Behavioral health issues may not have been the reason Fort Carson's soldiers committed violent crimes in 2008 and 2009, but behavioral health care didn't appear to have done enough to mitigate the causes.

The spate of violence around Fort Carson had resulted from a confluence of events, many of which had little to do with behavioral health care. But it's reasonable to wonder why the Army, which was seven years into an armed conflict that was obviously contributing to behavioral health problems on a large scale, did not have a ready supply of well-organized behavioral health professionals on every Army post. Where were the refined administrative resourcing and personnel processes to ensure that expert clinicians were hired and available? Where were the clinical programs delivering evidence-based care to soldiers returning from combat? Where were the strategies to form working relationships between leaders in the combat units and behavioral health clinicians to support soldiers with serious mental illnesses?

It turns out innovations were emerging at Army hospitals all over the world. Through trial and error, individual clinicians were finding better ways to deliver care to soldiers and their family members. For example, the team in Vicenza, Italy, had found a new way to increase soldiers' access to care by locating providers in small clinics in the unit areas. A group in Hawaii had developed a case management program that tracked each brigade's soldiers with serious mental illness to ensure they didn't fall out of treatment. In isolated locations throughout the Army, new clinical programs were emerging, insightful data were being collected, and clinical leaders were gaining efficiencies through better management techniques.

Unfortunately, these and other innovations were completely unknown to behavioral health staff in other locations who were not involved in their development. The clinical staff at Fort Carson, like the staff at most Army hospitals, had not heard about such advancements. The Army's health care system did not have a leadership team developing ways to identify the best practices popping up in its own hospitals. No one was building processes to replicate those best practices in its other hospitals and bring them together as part of a cohesive system of care. Local innovations remained confined to the posts where they were developed. Soldiers on any post other than the one where the innovations occurred could not benefit from them. When the system faltered, many soldiers dropped out of care and attempted to manage their symptoms on their own. In some instances—as in Colorado Springs—the consequences were catastrophic.

What happened in Colorado Springs was not isolated, and the Army's inability to provide needed mental health care was implicated further by incidents throughout the country. "Town by town across the United States," reported the *New York Times* at the beginning of 2008, "headlines have been telling similar stories. Lakewood, Washington: 'Family Blames Iraq After Son Kills Wife.' Pierre, South Dakota: 'Soldier Charged With Murder Testifies About Postwar Stress.' Colorado Springs: 'Iraq War Vets Suspected in Two Slayings, Crime Ring.'"[14]

The *Times* continued, fleshing out the references back to recent combat service:

> Individually, these are stories of local crimes, gut-wrenching postscripts to the war for the military men, their victims and their communities. Taken together, they paint the patchwork picture of a quiet phenomenon, tracing a cross-country trail of death and heartbreak.
>
> The *New York Times* found 121 cases in which veterans of Iraq and Afghanistan committed a killing in the United States, or were charged with one, after their return from war. In many of those cases, combat trauma and the stress of deployment—along with alcohol abuse, family discord and other attendant problems—appear to have set the stage for a tragedy that was part destruction, part self-destruction.
>
> Three-quarters of these veterans were still in the military at the time of the killing. More than half the killings involved guns, and the rest were stabbings, beatings, strangulations and bathtub drownings. Twenty-five offenders faced charges for murder, manslaughter or homicide for fatal car crashes resulting from drunken, reckless or suicidal driving.[15]

The rising prevalence of behavioral health conditions in soldiers was not a secret. As early as 2004, highly publicized, high-quality research on soldiers returning from deployments described a clear increase in the incidence of mental health conditions such as post-traumatic stress disorder, major depression, and generalized anxiety disorder.[16] The increase in demand for care was predictable, but as more and more soldiers sought it, they found that provider shortages and the use of treatments not based in sound evidence contributed to long waits for initial appointments, disrupted continuity, and reduced the effectiveness of the care once they finally received it.[17] A soldier entering a mental health clinic on a large Army post in 2008 routinely encountered an overcrowded waiting room with a line stretching out the door of the clinic. After waiting several hours to see a provider and complete the assessment, that soldier could expect to wait several weeks for a follow-up visit. Providers were simply overwhelmed with other cases.

As these sorts of stories spread, widespread shortfalls in clinical capacity began to garner the attention of Capitol Hill. In response, Congress provided supplemental funding that enabled the Army to expand significantly the behavioral health services available to soldiers and their family members. Army hospitals hired hundreds of additional behavioral health providers and support staff members. Between 2008 and 2012, the clinical staff grew from 2,721 clinical care providers to 3,731.[18] The number of soldier mental health appointments increased from 856,235 appointments to 1,320,555 over the same time.[19]

Much to the discouragement of leaders at all levels, however, the mental health of soldiers and their families did not appear to be improving. Outpatient clinics often failed to address completely soldiers' mental health conditions. The need for inpatient hospitalization for behavioral health problems continued to grow, from 178,225 bed days to 334,456 bed days in the same time period.[20] Media reports about inadequate behavioral health care services continued to pile up.

In 2009, a highly regarded civilian psychiatrist named Stephen Stahl visited Fort Hood in Killeen, Texas, to instruct clinicians there on current practices in the treatment of behavioral health conditions. He observed that the Army's mental health care system was "understaffed, under tremendous pressure, and near the breaking point."[21] Two years later, the *Pittsburgh Tribune-Review* reported that its own "nine-month investigation . . . buttressed by documents passed to the newspaper by soldiers and the Pentagon's Office of Wounded Warrior Care & Transition Policy . . . reveal[ed] an Army reeling from an epidemic of mental and behavioral health problems after nearly a decade of constant combat overseas."[22] The *Tribune-Review* recounted a litany of failures to provide needed behavioral health care services: "backed up" mental health clinics on and off post at Fort Drum in upstate New York; a program at Hawaii's Tripler Army Medical Center "not designed to be PTSD-specific" despite that "three out of every five Warrior

Transition soldiers brought there suffered from 'behavioral health issues'"; "only one Army mental health officer for every 265 cases" at the 25th Infantry Division's Schofield Barracks in Hawaii; and so on. And the article went on to reinforce the extent to which stigma was a problem.

Although related to many factors, some of which could not be directly affected by behavioral health care, more soldiers were committing suicide than since the wars began, and many of those soldiers had unaddressed mental health conditions. Soldiers commonly reported dissatisfaction with the care offered at Army hospitals and would leave treatment.[23] In 2012, the situation had deteriorated to the point where 184 soldiers committed suicide, the most since 2001.[24] Clearly, the investment in additional behavioral health resources was not paying off.

Frustrated leaders began to take a closer look at the Army's collection of behavioral health clinics and quickly discovered a major problem: unnecessary and unintended variance in how clinics were organized had created wide discrepancies in the type and quality of care they delivered. It was the same problem that JK's MIT team encountered. Each hospital's group of behavioral health clinics had been designed locally and was unique from all others. Most hospitals had developed new clinical programs that were intended to solve what were seen as the most pressing issues on that particular post. Some worked better than others, but as chapter 1 describes, the Army had not identified which were the *best* practices and replicated them in other hospitals.

Most hospitals had organized their behavioral health programs around massive centralized clinics that included dozens of providers practicing independently, not as part of a consistent multidisciplinary treatment team. Some programs used clinicians to conduct education and outreach into nonclinical settings, such as unit areas where soldiers would regularly gather. Other programs were tailored to individual clinicians' training or unique expertise, such as a handful that delivered biofeedback or animal-assisted therapy. Some posts had programs that offered care for family members, while others did not and referred all family members to the TRICARE network off the installation.

Programs to provide intensive treatment for soldiers with PTSD offer an excellent example. These programs are employed when soldiers' symptoms are severe enough to require more frequent appointments than can be delivered in a general outpatient behavioral health clinic, but not severe enough to require admission to an inpatient ward. At Fort Bliss in Texas, for instance, clinical psychologist John Fortunato designed an intensive treatment program delivered at the "Restoration and Resilience Center," named for the program. Fortunato was also a Vietnam veteran and a Benedictine monk, and his unique program—which included new office space and multiple therapeutic approaches—was well received by soldiers and senior Army leaders. During a 2008 visit, General George Casey, the Army chief of staff, praised the program and called for it to be replicated at other Army posts.[25]

While the program clearly filled an unmet need at Fort Bliss, it was also extremely resource- and personnel-intensive to run. Amid a national shortage of behavioral health providers that was particularly acute in the city of El Paso, where Fort Bliss is located, hospital leaders were forced to leave other needed positions vacant to run the Restoration and Resilience Center. The program also reflected Dr. Fortunato's unique talent; as General Casey articulated, "Unfortunately, you can't package John Fortunato and move him around and it really takes someone with that passion to drive these kinds of operations."[26]

Other Army hospitals grappling with the same problems developed different approaches to offer intensive outpatient treatment for soldiers with PTSD, often based on the personalities of the providers who worked there. At Fort Hood, also in Texas, the hospital developed an extensive program that incorporated a wide range of complementary and alternative treatment approaches, such as massage, reiki/bioenergy therapies, and tai chi. But space constraints made it impossible to expand the program, and the waiting times for new patients to begin the program grew to more than a year.[27]

At Landstuhl Regional Medical Center in Germany, the largest military hospital outside the continental United States, behavioral health care providers designed their own eight-week treatment program called "Evolution" that included whatever types of treatment the staff thought might work. As the chief of the Division of Behavioral Health, Dr. Daphne Brown, explained, "I am a great believer in the kitchen sink, meaning I throw in everything, including the kitchen sink, and something will stick." That included "all the evidence-based treatment for PTSD that we know about."[28]

Even though each of these local programs showed promising results, the variation, which in many cases stemmed from the personalities involved in developing or leading the efforts, meant that only the soldiers who happened to be assigned to a given post were benefiting from the best program. Soldiers at other posts were receiving less than optimal care.

In addition to divergence between the clinical programs delivering care to patients, critical processes within behavioral health clinics also varied. For instance, each hospital designed its own process for determining which patients may be at the highest risk for suicide and the procedures required to deliver care to this vulnerable group. Some facilities used validated screening instruments to ask their patients about suicidal thinking, while others relied solely on their clinicians' judgment. Some, but not all, required weekly follow-up for patients that were considered to be "high risk" for suicide. Some employed case managers to coordinate care for this group, while others required that the providers perform that function themselves.

Which method was the most effective at retaining patients in care and preventing suicide attempts? Most hospitals used the process they had developed locally because they were unaware of those developed at other facilities. The system did not have a mechanism for comparing facilities' approaches to determine which worked best.

Data collection also varied significantly between hospitals. Basic data, such as number of appointments and workload, as measured through RVUs, were consistently aggregated and reported in all hospitals.[29] But other more informative data, such as wait times for appointments or patient clinical improvements, either were not collected at all or, when they were, suffered from data quality problems that prevented comparisons across the system. Very few hospitals had the ability to turn their existing data into usable measures of efficiency or effectiveness. Many of those that did used locally developed formulas or tools that frequently depended on manual data entry and were kept on local spreadsheets. This variance confounded early attempts at analysis and made systematic improvement impossible.

These shortcomings did not escape the notice of the most senior Army leaders. General Peter W. Chiarelli, then the vice chief of staff of the US Army, more than once described the state of the Army's mental health care system as a field with "a thousand flowers blooming."[30] It wasn't meant as a compliment. He was expressing the frustration of nonmedical leaders across the Army. Mental health problems were negatively affecting their soldiers, their soldiers' families, and their units' ability to achieve its mission to fight and win wars in Iraq and Afghanistan. The primary system for addressing those problems, mental health clinics in Army hospitals, varied from post to post, provided inconsistent care, and made it harder for them to lead their soldiers successfully.

Despite growing experience with mental health issues from the ongoing wars, decades of military psychiatric experience from prior conflicts, and Congress allocating almost $200 million in annual supplemental funds beginning in 2007 specifically for psychological health, the Army by 2011 still had no consistently effective system for providing mental health care for soldiers stationed on its posts around the world.[31]

Chapter 3

ORGANIZING A LEARNING HEALTH CARE SYSTEM

When issues rise to, but are not addressed at, the system level, they persist and often get worse.

Sergeant Anderson returned from Afghanistan after a deployment that included surviving a Taliban ambush that killed four younger soldiers. Something had gone terribly wrong, and he could not get it out of his head that he was responsible—although his commander at the small forward operating installation outside Kabul had assured him that his actions saved many other lives that day. But after several sleepless weeks, he returned home to a stateside Army post and made a difficult decision to try to get some help.

His post had a small satellite behavioral health care clinic associated with the large Army hospital about twenty miles away, which required a drive that could take up to an hour in heavy traffic. The large majority of soldiers and their families lived near the satellite clinic, but most of the providers lived near the main hospital—which was where they preferred to see patients. The actual clinical services available in the satellite clinic were few and did not include the intensive treatment for PTSD Sergeant Anderson needed.

Like other patients, Sergeant Anderson had to make the drive to the main hospital for almost all of his appointments. And also like large numbers of patients, Sergeant Anderson dropped out of care after two weeks because he grew concerned that the long absences from work, about half a day a couple of times per week, were negatively affecting how his supervisors viewed his performance.

The hospital commander saw the numbers and knew this was a problem that wasn't going to get better. He directed the behavioral health leaders in his hospital to consider expanding the services available at the satellite location by shifting additional providers to the post itself, where the large majority of soldiers lived and worked. Within just a few days, the commander received a long list of reasons why it couldn't be done. The entire leadership of the behavioral health team claimed that it would have a detrimental effect on the clinic's efficiency. Internship and residency training programs would fall apart. And forget about provider retention if our people have to drive all the way to the post, they argued. Ultimately, they insisted, such a change would degrade care overall. Who would want that? they asked.

What the Army needed was a sober analysis of the problem, a review of the administrative data to account for the clinical considerations raised by the hospital's behavioral health leaders and solutions that addressed their concerns. But who could do that? The Army didn't have a team at a higher level of the organization equipped for such a task.

The commander was stuck and couldn't make the major changes to behavioral health care that he desired.

The Army lacked an empowered group of full-time professionals at the top of the system to guide the development of a true system of care and resolve problems plaguing leaders at each of its hospitals. At the system level, Army medicine relied on a group of senior officers in each major professional area—psychiatry, psychology, and social work—to be part-time consultants, primarily responsible for advancing the interests of their professional group. They had full-time jobs elsewhere in the enterprise, and when working on system-wide issues had no dedicated staff, such as expert clinicians, analysts, administrators, or resource managers. No one had the task of managing behavioral health care as a whole.

The vacuum created by the lack of a fully formed clinical team functioning within the Army medical headquarters was filled by the best efforts of leaders at each local hospital. For example, because no group of experts existed to compare hospitals' high-risk patient policies, determine which ones worked the best, and disseminate them to all other hospitals, each hospital published its own. Analytic experts did not work closely with clinical experts on a regular basis and therefore did not understand how hospital-level clinical leaders could use data to manage their clinics better. Instead, administrators in many hospitals developed their own technical methods for collecting and comparing data. For example, absent a *system* tool for easily monitoring the efficiency of each provider (as defined by the number of RVUs per month), hospitals had to devise their own local tools—with various levels of success. The lack of communication, common metrics, and standards prevented most hospitals from learning from the experiences of others, further exacerbating the problem of unnecessary variance across the system.

Three related issues were primarily responsible for the lack of a system-level leadership team. First, the culture and leadership philosophy within Army Medicine emphasized the authority of the local hospital commander and his/her subordinate leaders to design and execute health care. The idea was informed by the prevailing leadership philosophy within the broader Army, known as Mission Command, which cast the commander in charge of a specific mission as the most critical decision maker. That commander was therefore granted the greatest authority. When applied to the Army health care system, though, this left local hospital leaders with minimal guidance from system-level leaders about key issues, such as the design of new behavioral health clinics intended to meet the growing need for care—something exacerbated in a time of rapidly increasing complexity. As Patricia D. Horoho, 43rd Army surgeon general and commanding general of the US Army Medical Command (since retired), put it at the time, Army Medicine was functioning as a sort of "holding company," with system leaders invested in, but infrequently directing, local hospital operations, and in which local policy making and data collection, decentralized support services, and unique processes were the norm.[1]

Second, mental health care had not traditionally been viewed as an Army priority. Much more attention was given to other clinical areas before the wars in Iraq and Afghanistan. Trauma care was almost always viewed as much more critical to the Army's combat mission, and primary care was more relevant to keeping soldiers healthy enough to fight. And mental health providers rarely held influential senior leadership positions.

As an indication of the low priority in many Army hospitals, the mental health clinics were directed to operate out of space previously used by other clinical services. For example, one Army hospital used recently vacated inpatient internal medicine wards for its outpatient mental health clinic. The space had never been intended for mental health care and lacked group therapy rooms, two-way mirrors for observation and training new clinicians, and other features vital to providing services patients needed.

Finally, there was the lack of integration between the professional groups that made up mental health itself. From the system to the clinic level, psychiatrists, psychologists, and clinical social workers separated themselves by their disciplines—a problem that William Menninger had pointed out during his time on active duty during World War II.[2] At the system level, the specialty-specific consultants had influence only over those officers within their professional area. Their primary mission was to develop the careers of their officers and further the interests of their specialty within the Army and beyond. None of the three leaders could change a policy if it affected clinicians in another discipline, which effectively meant that no one could make the much-needed changes to close gaps in the system.

At the local level, most Army hospitals were divided into departments or services of psychiatry, psychology, and social work, each discipline with its own chief who managed a clinic independent from the other disciplines, referring patients back and forth when needed. In some instances, leaders worked well together to minimize the inconvenience and risk for patients as they attempted to receive therapy in one clinic, medications in another, and social interventions in a third. Gaps and redundancies between each discipline's clinical operations were, unfortunately, more typical.

Often, patients themselves were unsure of where to begin to access care because the process differed on each post. And many primary care providers did not know where to send a patient with depressive symptoms in need of a specialty evaluation. To the psychology clinic? The psychiatry clinic?

For example, a primary care provider might refer a soldier to a psychology clinic for an evaluation for depression. The psychologist, after confirming the diagnosis, would again refer the patient, this time to the psychiatry clinic, for an evaluation to determine whether an antidepressant medication might be helpful. That soldier would have been better served if the psychologist had consulted with a psychiatrist working in the same clinic and with whom she shared all patients in need of medication. Furthermore, treatment for an alcohol use disorder, support from the Family Advocacy Program, and other common clinical services all required separate referrals, more waiting, and new evaluations. In many cases, the multiple providers never met in person or even spoke by phone to discuss the nuances of a soldier's treatment, relying instead on reading each other's notes in the health record.

Disputes often erupted when leaders were forced to work together, such as to determine call schedules and emergency room coverage. In one infamous example, an intense disagreement broke out between departments of psychiatry and psychology at a large Army medical center. So much bitterness had been created over a long history of parochial disagreements that staff could not even work together to check patients in for appointments. So, they "solved" the problem by placing a large piece of colored tape down the middle of the front desk and declaring that psychology staff and patients would stay on one side of the line and psychiatry staff and patients on the other!

The front desk is an extreme example, but without a sufficient local leadership structure to resolve problems over things as trivial as pens and pencils, it's no wonder clinical operations were stovepiped and isolated. Collaboration between clinicians treating the same patients was inconsistent and treatment plans were often uncoordinated.

The persistent division between professional groups impaired young officers' leadership development just as much as it imperiled efficient and effective patient care. Most career-minded providers viewed their professional aspirations along the lines of their specific specialty. Psychologists strove to lead psychology clinics and psychology departments, and ultimately to serve as the consultant for psychology to the surgeon general. Psychiatrists and social workers did the same. At each level, each officer would lead only a slice of the personnel and resources required to treat mental health conditions adequately, which should include the participation of all specialties. As a result, few clinicians developed into leaders interested in or capable of providing oversight of behavioral health as a whole.

This suboptimal situation hummed along for decades without senior medical leaders fully understanding the problem. As long as the number of patients seeking care remained relatively low, the professional divisions could be navigated and the local disputes tolerated. But the wars in Iraq and Afghanistan and the sharp increase in demand for mental health care they spurred blew that up. As more soldiers and their family members experienced symptoms of mental illness and attempted to initiate care, the Army behavioral health system's flaws were exposed. Negative attention from the media and members of Congress and a strong desire to do better for Army beneficiaries struggling with mental illness rapidly raised the priority senior leaders gave to behavioral health. It was the beginning of the Army's pursuit of a learning mental health system: senior medical leaders grasped that major changes were necessary, that they would take a long time, and that a group of experienced mental health leaders would be needed at the system level to accomplish them.

Building a Mental Health Leadership Structure

While the struggles within Army behavioral health care were particularly formidable, they were not completely unique. Reducing unwanted variance at the clinical level had also challenged primary care, surgery, and musculoskeletal care. Realizing that significant changes were needed to improve care in almost all areas of Army hospital performance, the surgeon general in 2012 made a major alteration to the governing philosophy that had guided Army Medicine for decades, if not longer. Determining that systematic changes to all hospitals would be impossible without fundamental changes in how the Army operated its hospitals, she announced that Army hospitals would henceforth adhere to the Operating Company Model (OCM), an approach that emphasized shared organizational values and process standardization around proven best practices. It shifted more authority for policy making, strategic planning, and program development to the headquarters level and away from individual hospitals. The OCM provided a critical centralizing influence that balanced the principles of Mission Command.

The action Horoho took built on preliminary steps that had begun to unfold as far back as 2007, motivated in large part by the congressional funding increase. A small group of people at Army Medicine headquarters had begun to think through how to manage various parts of behavioral health and solve some of the problems, even if at first somewhat haphazardly. They wanted to make sure not to waste the extra money that had been allocated. This group grew, but without the support of an overarching philosophy to guide active leadership engagement throughout the Army's medical system.

As Army Medicine shifted to the OCM, it needed a structure to manage each major clinical area and link the system-level leadership team with the clinical teams operating in clinics across the enterprise. The surgeon general selected the service line model and established Behavioral Health (the newly accepted Army term for mental health) as the first clinical service line.[3] The system-level component of the Behavioral Health Service Line (BHSL) would operate from the combined headquarters of the Office of the Surgeon General and the US Army Medical Command, building on the nucleus that had first emerged in 2007 and consolidating all behavioral health actions, authorities, expertise, funding, and analysis in a single, cohesive team. The personnel included a group of experienced clinical leaders, administrators, and analysts already working within the headquarters; a prescient clinical leader who had anticipated that a new team would be needed to improve behavioral health care throughout the Army had formed the team. Other personnel were reassigned from positions in Army hospitals or newly hired. The clinicians represented all clinical specialties within mental health and were organized under a single chief selected by the surgeon general. The Army now had a group of dedicated professionals empowered by the operating company model to make system-wide changes to improve mental health care.

Clinical service lines are nothing new outside of the Army; they've been used for several decades. They may be best described as health care units organized around the clinical needs of a group of patients, not the professional background of the clinical staff. Service lines can also be viewed as the management-level version of integrated practice units, the multidisciplinary foundation of value-based care, because they facilitate measurement and accountability of patient-centered processes, outcomes, and costs.[4] In the Army's version, the hospital commander functions like a chief executive officer and is responsible for all care delivered in that facility. However, enterprise-wide standards, processes, programs, and policies that govern behavioral health care come from the service line leadership team at the health system level in the Office of the Surgeon General (see figure 3.1). This arrangement, sometimes called "matrixed," allows for the thoughtful distribution of authority between system-level service line leaders and hospital-level leadership teams.[5]

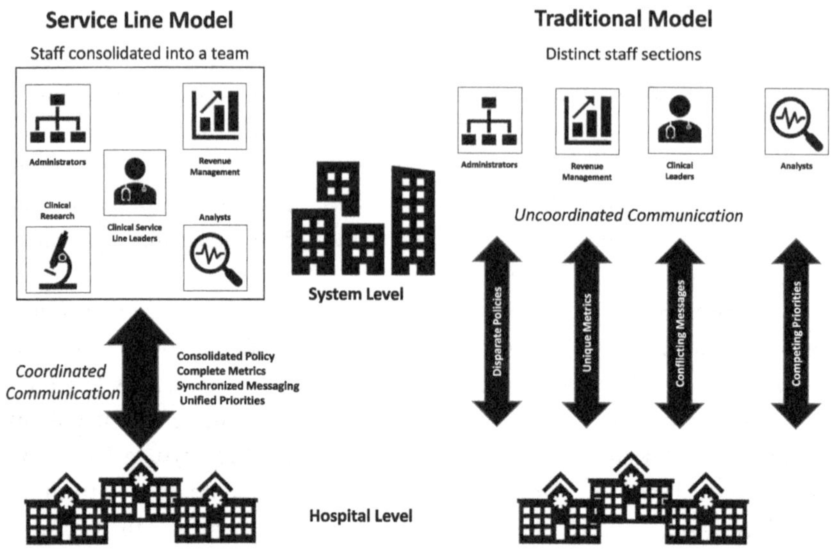

FIGURE 3.1. Unified service line leadership model vs. traditional model

Army medical leaders and clinicians, however, did not uniformly accept the shift to the OCM and the creation of the service line. While most hospital-level leaders were somewhat wary, they appreciated that the enterprise had assembled clinically informed teams whose role was to support local leaders as they improved care. A minority saw service lines as an intrusion on their authority and independence and resisted. It fell to service line leaders operating at the system level to build trust with local leaders.

The service line team alleviated local leaders' concerns primarily by demonstrating that the service line would help local leaders solve practical problems. During a scheduled visit to a large Army hospital in 2016, the chief of the service line was pulled aside by the hospital commander. The frustrated hospital executive told him that he wanted to increase the number of patients his facility treated on the inpatient behavioral health ward. However, the chief of his department of behavioral health refused to do so, citing patient safety concerns. The service line chief agreed to look into the issue. Later that day, the service line chief spoke with the department chief. "The hospital commander doesn't really get it," he was told. The chief accused the commander of "undervaluing" the contributions of the behavioral health providers. "I had some providers on staff we could not do without," he told the service line chief. "I wanted to keep them. But when I asked for retention bonuses a few weeks ago to keep them on, the commander refused. They're all gone now," having left for higher-paying positions at other hospitals, "and there are consequences." It wasn't too difficult for the service line chief to figure out that the department chief's refusal to increase the inpatient ward capacity was aimed first and foremost at sending a message to the hospital commander about his decision. Of course, a stalemate didn't serve patient needs.

Service line leaders intervened and broke the impasse. They recommended ways—based on practices they had observed in other Army hospitals—to free inpatient providers from several time-consuming duties, such as emergency department consultations, so they would have sufficient time to treat additional patients on the ward. They also lent legitimacy to the department chief's complaint about the commander's lack of support for retention bonuses by showing the commander that similar bonuses were being paid by other Army hospitals.

The intervention worked. Capacity on the ward was expanded—albeit somewhat reluctantly on the part of the provider staff—which pleased the hospital commander. And the commander agreed to look more favorably on future requests for retention bonuses for behavioral health providers. Over time, trust between service line and hospital leaders grew and positive working relationships were established with almost all hospital leaders.

The BHSL at the system level incorporated all behavioral health-related personnel actions and authorities into its organization. All other sections within the headquarters and related to behavioral health, such as social work services and the Family Advocacy Program (the Army equivalent of Child Protective Services), were also integrated into the BHSL team. This was key: the Army saw the limitations of the "center of excellence" models that were in use at the Department of Defense level and in other large organizations such as the Veterans Administration and opted instead to place its system-level behavioral health leadership team directly within its headquarters.

The Department of Defense's Centers of Excellence (DCoE) for Psychological Health and Traumatic Brain Injury, created in 2007, demonstrated the DoD's motivation to improve psychological health, but the problems that continued to plague military behavioral health care indicated that DCOE fell well short of its mission statement that it "assesses, validates, oversees, identifies, and facilitates prevention, resilience, screening, treatment, outreach, rehabilitation, and reintegration programs for PH and TBI to ensure the Department of Defense meets the needs of the nation's warriors, families, and military communities."[6]

The service line model offered several advantages over one or more centers of excellence. It allowed the leadership team to create a single vision for behavioral health care, establish priorities for resourcing, and ensure that leaders at local hospitals knew who to reach out to with questions, problems, or suggestions. The unified approach enabled cohesive and coordinated actions by system-level experts to help local leaders address priority issues.

The use of centers of excellence locates resources and personnel with expertise in a specific sub-area, such as PTSD, *away* from the primary clinical leadership team—creating barriers between that knowledge and the mechanisms to disseminate it throughout the system. In contrast, the Army's service line model gave behavioral health leaders full responsibility for all aspects of soldiers', family members', and other beneficiaries' behavioral health care. Clinical experts in important areas, such as PTSD, domestic violence, and, eventually, substance use disorders, were built directly in to the staff of the BHSL team.

As system-level behavioral health leaders began to form a leadership team, early experiences helped them learn which capabilities would be needed to transform the Army's behavioral health care system.

Key Functional Areas

Four key functional areas emerged and were incorporated into the enterprise-level team in the Office of the Surgeon General. The first concerned *service line leadership*. Leaders would have as their primary role to ensure that behavioral health teams functioned efficiently and effectively so learning could take place at every level. The Army found it critical that the service line leader be a clinician, because clinicians are most thoroughly grounded in patient care and can most readily relate to providers' experiences in delivering care. Clinical leaders would also ensure that executive medical and nonmedical leaders learn about the behavioral health care system. This aspect would be important because informed executive leaders can best direct resources and focus the entire system's attention on the most relevant and pressing issues.

Second, *clinical program management* emerged as a key functional area for the enterprise-level team. As the behavioral health leadership identified major areas of the behavioral health care delivery system that needed standardization and improvement, it would identify a corresponding best practice in use in the field. Examples of programmatic best practices included intensive outpatient treatment programs, Embedded Behavioral Health clinics, and Child and Family Behavioral Health clinics. To support implementation across all hospitals and improve performance over time, the Army created clinical program management teams comprised of clinicians and administrators with direct experience in the program being replicated.

Clinical program managers also created learning opportunities for local leaders engaged in executing the program. For example, the Embedded Behavioral Health program managers held monthly forums via teleconference to discuss problems arising at the local level and share strategies for overcoming them. Program managers engineered solutions for problems that could not be solved locally, such as creating standard position descriptions for all hospitals to use when hiring new staff. Program managers also traveled to many locations to train staff, work through facility issues, and reinforce the hard work being done by local clinical leaders. They served to focus the resources available at the system level on priority programs and facilitated learning by local leaders to improve performance continually.

The primary job of the *analytics* component of the team, which was the third functional area that emerged, is to transform raw data into useable forms, such as metrics. For example, the utility at the system level of measurement-based care, a major component of a learning behavioral health system, depends on analysts' ability to aggregate and make meaning out of millions of data points generated by patient and provider input. Analytics takes the digital representation of the care itself and presents it to clinicians, administrators, and leaders. Analysts also assist service line leaders by using data to respond to questions from executive leaders and other stakeholders.

Finally, the executive-level team would have to make sure there was *fiscal and administrative oversight* as a functional capability. Administrators at the hospital level have key roles in health care operations, especially when change is occurring. The BHSL teams included personnel with administrative expertise to ensure that changes on the clinical side were matched on the administrative side. For example, as new clinical programs were created and replicated, a series of administrative actions were required to ensure that clinical personnel and workload were accounted for, front desk staff were trained to perform new tasks, and funding was properly allocated. Clinical leaders often have a poor understanding of the importance and complexity of administrative functions, but seasoned administrators operating as part of the enterprise-level team are invaluable in communicating with administrators at the local level to guide change efforts. In addition, administrators with experience in resource management were critical in developing funding models, including incentives that aligned with best clinical practices. Table 3.1 summarizes these functional areas and their connection to *learning* as part of a behavioral health system.

BHSL leaders quickly identified that the large number of mental health programs that had been developed by each Army hospital created a major source of unnecessary variance.[7] In conjunction with the US Army Public Health Command and systems engineers at the Massachusetts Institute of Technology, the BHSL mapped the collection of clinical BH programs in use at Army hospitals to find redundancies and inefficiencies and to identify innovative clinical programs that

TABLE 3.1 Key capabilities and functions

CAPABILITY	FUNCTIONS	ROLE IN LEARNING
Service line leadership	Integrate and lead the team	Oversee total system learning Ensure senior leaders and other key stakeholders learn about the behavioral health system
Clinical program management	Support the implementation and clinical operations of major standardized programs	Ensure learning within each clinical program
Analytics	Produce data, including clinical outcomes drawn from measurement-based care; respond to questions using objective information	Generate data for all to use as a basis for learning
Administrative and fiscal oversight	Align nonclinical data systems, such as workload and personnel accounting, with clinical program operations	Ensure learning by local administrators

represented best practices.[8] A group of clinical programs that successfully demonstrated promising outcomes and filled a critical need were found and put on a path for replication throughout other Army hospitals over the coming period.

But to replicate clinical programs across the enterprise, the Army had to develop behavioral health leadership teams at all levels of the system.

Local Leadership

Integrating the professional mental health groups in its hospitals and clinics was one of the BHSL leadership's most important early actions. The divisions between psychology, psychiatry, and clinical social work were inhibiting learning at the clinic and hospital levels. The BHSL issued a policy in 2013 that expressly prohibited Army hospitals from organizing solely around the professional discipline of a group of providers, requiring instead that they integrate all clinical mental health operations under one department, led by a single chief. The policy organized hospital staff into clinical teams based on patient needs, provided new leadership opportunities across disciplines, and reduced parochial infighting. It outlined a process and qualification guidelines by which hospital commanders should select the most qualified person for the chief position, who could be a clinician from any clinical background. For the first time in many locations, providers who had not had the opportunity to serve in interdisciplinary leadership roles, particularly psychologists and clinical social workers with outstanding leadership skills, took charge of entire departments of behavioral health. The changes reiterated that the needs of the patients were now the central organizing principle within Army behavioral health care.

This large-scale change, however, didn't go smoothly at all locations. At one large Army hospital, for instance, the chief of psychology voiced deep concerns to his hospital commander about making the change to an interdisciplinary department. He had spent several years constructing a large department with several niche programs, such as a unique approach to smoking cessation. He was worried about losing the programs.

Those niche programs, while effective, had a problem: they were very inefficient. They required large numbers of clinical staff while providing care to only small numbers of patients. There was plenty of evidence from elsewhere that the same services could be provided more efficiently using other approaches—but at this hospital the approaches had been built around the particular interests of a few providers, whom the chief of psychology was also concerned about losing. The chief had maintained these programs despite the fact that staffing shortages in his department and in psychiatry and social work were impairing other higher-demand clinical services, such as outpatient care for soldiers with depression and PTSD.

The hospital commander called in the system-level team for an on-site visit to analyze the chief of psychology's concerns in detail and present a plan for the best way to consolidate the three departments into one and arrange the clinical staff to deliver the best care. The system-level service line team spent three weeks dissecting the hospital's three-department structure, mapping out lines of authority, analyzing workload, and identifying gaps in care delivery. The team assembled a plan to consolidate the specialty-specific departments into one and showed the commander how that would better align the clinical staff with the highest-demand services. The niche programs would be absorbed into larger, enterprise-wide ones, and more soldiers with the most serious conditions would get better care. His concerns addressed, the hospital commander went forward with the plan to merge the three departments and realign the clinical staff to areas of highest need.

Throughout the Army, a series of transformative changes resulted in a common set of clinical programs operated by multidisciplinary groups of clinicians managed through a unified system of clinical experts—a first for the Army. The transformation of the Army's behavioral health clinics had begun with the creation of a leadership structure that stretched from the system to the clinic level. Leaders represented all professional disciplines within mental health and included analysts, administrators, and resource management experts—all critical to building the learning loops to be described in later chapters. The team helped develop the management processes to oversee other large components of health care.

Senior medical leaders empowered behavioral health leaders to assess the care being provided across the enterprise and make radical changes wherever necessary to reduce unwanted variance.

The Challenge of Delivering Mental Health Care

Delivering quality mental health care in one facility, let alone multiple locations, is no easy task. Nearly every comprehensive examination of mental health care in the United States in the past two decades has concluded that it falls far short of basic benchmarks and must make major, fundamental changes to achieve high-quality care on a consistent basis. For example, the Institute of Medicine (now National Academy of Medicine) has called for major and ambitious modifications to broad areas at multiple levels, such as integration of mental and physical health care, increasing resources, improving measurement, and enhancing training.[9] Health care systems must do more than make one-time changes to improve quality; instead, they must build systems that learn and perpetually improve over time—which often requires extensive changes to information technology and in the culture, to name just a few.[10] Taken together, these actions amount to transforming how mental health care systems operate, from the C-suite to the clinic.

Successfully navigating the twofold challenge of expanding any health system, mental health or otherwise, while simultaneously transforming it, depends on an organization's ability to understand and manage variance—intentional and unintentional—across its clinical delivery locations, both in terms of how things are done, such as deviations from a standard of practice or a specific care plan, and outcomes such as differences in personnel costs, efficiency (as indicated by RVU production per provider), clinical outcomes, and patient satisfaction. The differences in clinical operations between outpatient clinics and inpatient wards performing similar functions for similar patient populations can be immense and can impair the performance of the system as a whole. When a process varies, the outcomes will also vary.

Of course, not all patients are the same, and the practice of medicine cannot be reduced to an algorithm. The key for health care system leadership teams is to determine whether the variance between clinics, hospitals, and other entities is intentional to benefit patients or the unintended consequence of the system falling short.

Intentional variance is when the clinical team decides to tailor its actions to the patient—such as creating a unique treatment plan—because of comorbid conditions (that is, the presence of additional diseases or disorders co-occurring with the primary disease or condition), access to transportation, willingness to participate in particular treatment options, or other reasons. For example, treatment teams may forego using psychotherapy to treat a particular patient's depression, even if it is evidence-based, because that patient specifically states that he does not wish to participate in it and cannot be convinced otherwise. Instead, the team may use medications only.

Unintentional variance occurs when the treatment team cannot or chooses not to employ the best practice for the patient. (Throughout this book, when we use the term "best practice," we are referring to a set of interrelated work activities repeatedly utilized by individuals or groups that a body of knowledge demonstrates will yield an optimal result.) If a patient presents to an outpatient mental health clinic with symptoms of major depression, for instance, he should receive an assessment and treatment options that are consistent with professional guidelines and organizational standards and delivered in the most efficient possible manner. Unintentional variance would be the failure to offer evidence-based psychotherapy that is consistent with clinical practice guidelines because a provider has not been trained to deliver it. Another example is not offering case management services for complex or high-risk patients because there is no care coordinator, even though the health care system has a policy stating that clinics will hire one. Unintentional variance also occurs when one element of the health care system has identified a best practice and is using it to improve care for its patients, but other elements of the system are unaware of the practice or unable to institute it. It happens frequently: one clinic solves a problem, but other clinics aren't informed about or can't implement the solution.

Unintentional variance runs rampant when the system cannot effectively measure and manage key components of the episode of care, such as ensuring its providers are trained on evidence-based treatments and monitoring each patient's progress with common clinical outcome tools. Absent skilled oversight and active support, clinical care diverges from the standard, and the risk for adverse outcomes increases.

Learning health care systems encourage and support intentional variance while identifying and minimizing unintentional variance. Clinically informed leadership teams, though, can identify best practices in the field, modify training and policy, and generate effective tools to support clinicians. In the end, patients experience more consistent care delivered through best practices according to prevailing standards. Clinically focused leadership teams at all levels reduce variance through a constant process of assessing and improving care across time and space. They simultaneously support their own clinical staff and overcome the inherent resistance to change while maintaining a clear focus on the ultimate goal of improving the health of the patient.

Unfortunately, many systems do not have an adequate clinical leadership structure in place to make the changes necessary to create and maintain an effective mental health system. Why do so many systems lack effective leaders in mental health care? Some argue that leadership training and development in mental health professional education programs has lagged other medical professions, or that mental health professionals are more inclined than most to avoid leadership roles. While these are both challenges, neither is easily addressed by most health care delivery systems that operate beyond the academic setting, and they can be overcome by well-structured systems. Three other problems that impair effective mental health leadership are even more relevant, but can be addressed by any health care system: the low priority given to mental health care within an organization; the lack of integration between professional groups within mental health and between mental and physical health teams; and overly decentralized decision-making authority. Many of these issues also confound attempts to improve physical health care, and the Army's experience confronting them within behavioral health care may be informative for those working to do a better job developing clinical leaders.

Lessons beyond the Army

The challenges the Army faced, and the solutions the Army developed, are relevant to other health care systems as they work to deliver excellent care within a consistent patient experience at numerous locations.

A main lesson from the Army's experience is that health care systems must minimize unintentional variance and promote and learn from intentional variance. That can happen only if a learning system is enabled system-wide, which requires processes and critical elements that are the subject of the chapters to come. At the overall level, the Army learned that the key to successful clinical operations across an organization is a fully established and empowered behavioral health leadership structure operating at all levels of the system.

How can leaders determine whether they have a sufficient behavioral health leadership structure in place to understand variance, learn from its best practices, and improve performance? The answer lies in integration, leadership balance, and priorities.

The Army found major barriers to learning within behavioral health care because it did not organize its professional groups in a manner consistent with how care was delivered. Collaboration between psychiatry, psychology, and clinical social workers were required to achieve the standard of care at the clinical level, but department boundaries prevented individual providers from effective interfacing for the benefit of the patient. For example, psychiatrists and psychotherapists couldn't developing consistent working relationships and coordinate care because they did not attend the same meetings, adhere to the same policies, or strive for the same metrics. Part of the solution was found in *horizontal integration*—the process of organizing all clinical and nonclinical behavioral health staff into a single department to create clinical teams based on patient needs, not the diplomas on the providers' walls. That eliminated most artificial hurdles. To be sure, certain activities must have a discipline-specific component—for example, peer review, graduate professional education, and some professional development—but the care delivery structure and the teams that lead it must represent all professional groups. With the patient at the center, teamwork and communication between professionals, which are fundamental components of learning, become logical and expected.

A few important questions can shed light for other health care systems on their degree of horizontal integration. Do clinics include professionals from all disciplines who are required to meet the standard of care for the disorders they treat? Do those professionals work with the same group of people from other disciplines? For example, does a psychologist work with the same psychiatrist when her patients are in need of psychopharmacotherapy, or does she have to find a different psychiatrist with whom to collaborate for each patient? Can leaders at the clinic, hospital, or system level come from any professional discipline, or are top leadership positions only for certain groups? At the system level, are all behavioral health–related groups organized under a single leader, or is expert knowledge sequestered away from the leadership teams engaged in system oversight, such as in "centers of excellence"?

Strictly horizontal integration, though, is insufficient—as the Army learned. *Vertical integration*—a clear connection between leadership teams at the clinic through system levels—is also critical to a strong leadership structure. The Army found that to drive system change and improve performance, system-level leaders must readily understand all aspects of the care delivered at the clinic level, including the administrative, technical, and resourcing requirements. Communication between clinics, hospitals, and system leaders was critical. In turn, the system-level team required the authority to provide guidance and issue policy all the way down to the clinical level.

Is a health care system sufficiently vertically integrated to support effective behavioral health leadership? Asking these questions will help to shed light. Is there an adequate leadership team at the clinic, hospital, and system levels? Are leadership teams led by clinicians? Do they include personnel with analytic, administrative, and resource management expertise? Do leaders across levels come together regularly to review performance, understand problems, develop solutions, and monitor changes?

The Army's experience clearly demonstrated that in addition to appropriate horizontal and vertical integration, influence and oversight from the system level was necessary to synchronize processes and improve outcomes across multiple hospitals. Without active engagement in the form of meetings, trainings, policies, and resourcing solutions, the system would have continued to foster unintentional variance. Senior health system leaders must create the expectation that their system-level behavioral health team represents them when creating standards, developing policy, and monitoring performance.

To accomplish this, the Army adopted the operating company model philosophy, which emphasized the importance of shared organizational values, centralized analysis of data, and a commitment to standardizing around best practices. Within that framework, the behavioral health team could readily identify and address the clinic-level problems that diminished performance. At the same time, system-level behavioral health leaders had to respect constraints experienced by local leaders and remain open to innovation.

All of this speaks to a *leadership philosophy that balances local management with system-level oversight*. Other health care systems can ask themselves whether their hospital-level leaders share the same goals and priorities as their system-level leaders. Do they see the system-level behavioral health team as a helpful, problem-solving entity? Are local leaders expected to structure behavioral health care in their facility according to system-wide best practices that may have been developed elsewhere? Do system-level teams respect local decision-making authority and appreciate the complexities involved in running behavioral health clinics?

The final lesson here is that *behavioral health must be a priority*. For the Army, it was a series of well-publicized crises that vaulted behavioral health into the forefront of organizational consciousness. Violence shook Army communities. Suicide rates increased. Readiness decreased. In response, leaders at all levels set new priorities to improve the care Army hospitals provided, including allocating additional resources, providing new clinic space, and shining a light on how effectively Army hospitals were providing care. Major changes that had once been thought impossible became a reality precisely because behavioral health became much more important to key stakeholders, such as members of Congress, Army generals, and hospital commanders.

The Army faced a public outcry. Other health care systems that do not have that same experience may not see mental health care as a priority. Contributing to the lack of attention, reimbursement rates for mental health care are low relative to other areas of medicine, and senior hospital and system leaders rarely come from the mental health disciplines. A lack of prioritization may manifest in many ways. Is adequate clinical space (such as within primary care clinics) allocated to behavioral health providers, even when inconvenient to other health care teams? Are behavioral health leaders involved in hospital and system-level decision-making meetings? Do senior system-level leaders personally engage to support their behavioral health leaders on contentious issues?

Ultimately, health care systems are judged by whether they consistently deliver effective care in an efficient manner across all treatment venues. A well-organized leadership structure enables the system to learn continually from variance and to control the variance that imperils consistently excellent care.

The Army received a crash course in improving and standardizing behavioral health care and found that the most important first step in establishing a learning organization was to create and empower clinical leadership teams from the clinic level up to the system level. By ensuring behavioral health is both horizontally and vertically integrated, supported by a philosophy that balances system goals with local needs, and regarded as a priority along with other areas of health care, other health care organizations can establish the conditions for optimal performance in all its care delivery locations, system-wide.

Chapter 4
FIVE LEVELS OF LEARNING

Specialist Johnson is in crisis when he is escorted into one of the behavioral health clinics on his Army post. His regular provider has a full schedule and cannot see him, so he is assigned to see the first available clinician. This provider knows absolutely nothing about his circumstances or his treatment plan. She takes a few minutes to look through Johnson's cumbersome medical record while he sits there waiting to talk with her, but that doesn't tell her enough to do anything more than a quick evaluation to ensure he is safe. She concludes that he is, telling the escort that Specialist Johnson poses no risk to himself or others and that he has been scheduled for a follow-up appointment the following week with his regular provider.

When Specialist Johnson returns to his unit, however, his commander is still worried. The commander has spoken with Johnson's immediate supervisor, who told him about the soldier's history of cutting behavior, his recent breakup with a longtime girlfriend, and his comments to buddies about how everything feels "empty." The commander immediately places Johnson on unit watch—which means the soldier is kept under a constant watchful eye and is accompanied by a more senior soldier wherever he goes. This continues until the follow-up appointment the next week. The result is to attach further stigma not only Specialist Johnson's own use of mental health care but also to the potential use by other members of his unit who might need it—after all, they are afraid they, too, may be subject to a unit watch. The episode also deteriorates the command team's trust in the clinic, because even though the provider had talked to the escort, she had not taken the time to gather the contextual information from the command team about Johnson's prior behaviors.

Specialist Johnson's story illustrates some of the limitations of a system in which providers have not and cannot learn about patients treated by other clinicians. The system was not designed to give providers the "time and space" they need, even to learn about potential at-risk patients with whom they may come in contact. This lack of protected time for providers to reflect on other patients, and space to share their lessons learned with clinician colleagues, results in knowledge gaps that can lead to adverse patient outcomes. And it speaks to a larger learning problem across the entire mental health care system.

The National Academy of Medicine prescribes a vision of a learning health care system (LHS) in which informatics, incentives, and culture are all aligned in a way that enables continuous improvement and innovation.[1] The core idea is that the vast amounts of data generated on every patient, during every clinical and nonclinical interaction, can be used to learn what works best for and will thus improve that patient's health outcomes. This learning can then be shared systematically across the LHS to improve overall performance.

Realizing this vision is at the very beginning stages, and there are few examples of large-scale learning health systems, let alone a learning *mental* health care system.[2] A recent series of workshops on building a national-scale LHS have argued that more research is needed to create a new science of learning systems.[3] In other words, there is no recipe to replicate.

As already described, the Army's mental health system prior to 2010 was organized anarchy. There were more than two hundred experiments being conducted across all thirty-four Army hospitals to find better approaches to meeting the changing mental health care needs of soldiers and their families. The learning from all these local experiments was distributed and often disconnected. It had to be systematized so the Army could determine what worked and then spread it across all Army hospitals. That required the Army to examine learning at five levels (shown in figure 4.1: as part of *patient care*; within a *clinic*; across clinics within a *hospital*; within the *health system* as a whole, including all providers, clinics, and hospitals; and from the *health care environment*).

The connection of learning within and across the levels resulted in the first large-scale learning mental health care system in the United States that, in turn, could create a consistent patient experience of care and improve patient outcomes. Let's take a closer look at each of these levels and the learning processes that unfold within each level.

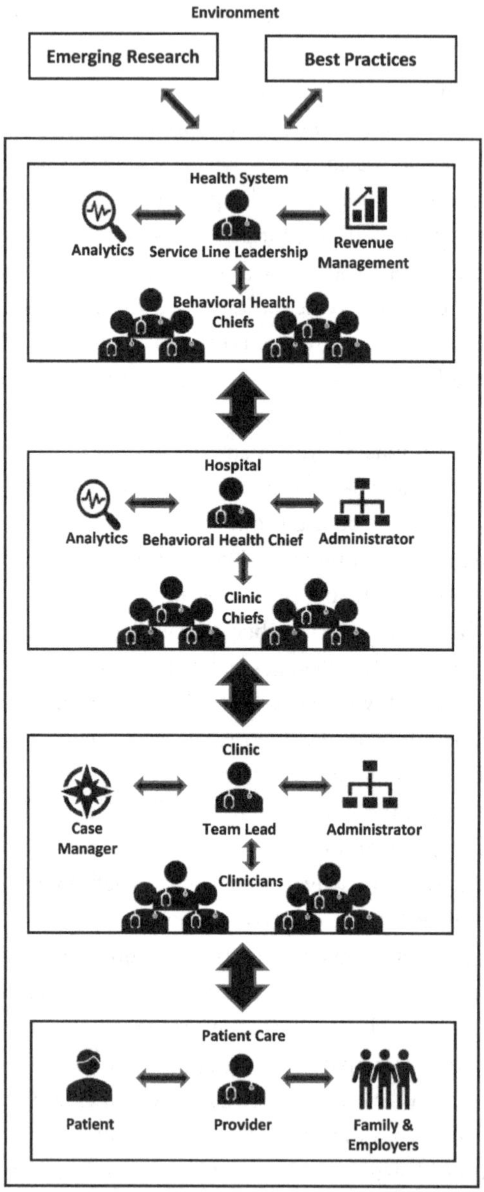

FIGURE 4.1. Five learning levels

Learning at the Patient-Care Level

Learning at the level of patient care is the foundation for any learning health care system. Unlike in other health care settings where a clinician can rely on laboratory tests, in individual or group settings patient-provider interactions are the main sources of information for clinical decision making in mental health care. At this level, the ways in which three particular processes unfold are closely linked to learning.

The first of these learning processes at the patient-care level concerns how providers keep up to date with their clinical skills, which may be routine. Learning happens when that process is not routine, but rather focuses on *improving and enhancing* provider clinical skills specifically to meet patient needs.

That wasn't happening consistently in the Army. Mental health care providers must improve their clinical skills to maintain their professional licensure and retain privileges to deliver care in any health care system.[4] The processes that *enhance clinical skills* include provider-driven continuing education, training in evidence-based treatment practices, and reflexive clinical practice. The first two are easier to implement than the third.

In the Army, the clinical skills of mental health care providers were assumed to be adequate based on their *academic training*. Specifically, that meant providers had graduated from professional society–certified clinical care programs and maintained their status as independently licensed practitioners in their chosen disciplines. Further, the Army used the fact that providers maintained their licenses as a proxy to determine whether clinical skills were sufficient to treat soldiers and family members—regardless of what they were being treated for or what that treatment might entail. That left the primary responsibility for enhancing clinical skills on individual providers, rather than it being an issue for the health system as a whole.

On top of that, soldiers had no way to know whether providers they were seeing were even using the therapies that made the most sense for their conditions. We spoke to soldiers at an Army post in 2011 about the quality of mental health care, and one young soldier told us, "I don't want to go mental health. There's a lovely lady there who tries to get me to play with figurines in a sandbox. How is that supposed to help me with my PTSD from the Iraq deployment?"

We were scheduled later that day to meet a clinician who wanted to share a unique practice she thought was a game changer for dealing with trauma. Guess what we saw when we walked into her office? A sand tray with a collection of figurines! There are legitimate arguments that a sensory-based approach such as sand tray therapy may be effective at treating trauma.[5] That clinician, however, had trained to work with children. She believed sandbox therapy would also be effective for soldiers, but it was not the recommended first-line treatment. No wonder the soldier was skeptical.

The second process at the patient-care level is about maintaining patients in care. Mental health care is rarely delivered in just one visit; most often, it requires continued interaction between patient and provider to realize sustained improvement in symptom reduction and health outcomes, and if a patient drops out of treatment, that cannot be accomplished. Learning happens when that process is focused on keeping patients *fully engaged* in their own care; patient engagement is a foundational element of any learning health care system.[6] At the patient-care level, engagement of patients in their own care is essential for effectively integrating their values, experiences, and perspectives into developing treatment plans and tracking patient progress toward recovery. Providers who engage patients in this way learn through real-time interactions with patients and through the retrospective review of case notes of prior interactions.

But just as with enhancing the clinical skills of providers, the Army—rather than taking active steps to ensure engagement—simply operated under the *assumption* that its independently licensed clinicians were able to engage their patients in care. That, however, was not the case. Instead, the Army's problem was soldiers *dropping out of care.*

Consider the earlier story of the sandbox. A soldier who wanted to get care for his combat PTSD did not perceive the treatment as being effective, so he stopped seeing the clinician. That provider was not able to engage that soldier in his own care.

When infantry soldiers were asked in a study why they dropped out of care, the common answers included insufficient time with providers, not liking the medications they had been offered, and not liking the talk therapy option.[7] More than half of the soldiers cited the occupational environment as a reason, too, specifically mentioning being too busy with work as well as the stigma associated with seeking mental health care.

Something a leader told us during a visit to Fort Bliss, Texas, really hit home about this link between the work and stigma. "For my soldier to go to mental health," he said,

> she would have to drive all the way to the hospital. We are at the other end of post. It takes forty-five minutes to drive to the hospital, even more time to find parking, and then the same amount of time to drive back to the soldiers' duty station. My soldier is essentially gone for half a day. Guess what? If that soldier is in an important job, everyone is asking questions. Where is that soldier? For my senior noncommissioned officers, there is the added challenge that they feel responsible for taking care

> of their own soldiers, and making sure they are trained for combat! They don't think they can make the time to get care for themselves!

The third process related to learning at the patient-care level concerns the environment for recovery. Learning happens when there is a conscious effort to shape the recovery environment—not only in the clinic but also beyond, through ongoing, appropriate engagement of family members and employers. The Army was largely failing at this, too.

Part of that failure stemmed from a problem found throughout the Army: the timely HIPAA-compliant sharing of information between providers and commanders was, at best, ad hoc and unsystematic.[8] When we spoke to command teams, they typically told us that providers didn't share any information with them, even though required to do so, and that providers never reached out to verify the stories they heard from their soldier patients or to discuss the occupational context of a soldier's treatment.

How does this affect a soldier's work environment? "If I know what that soldier needs," one commander explained, "I can make sure that I can help that soldier—even if it means taking that soldier to the field without a firing pin in their weapon. That way, the soldier is still part of the unit, and no one needs to know why the soldier is not in the field with them! But I can't do that because the behavioral health provider didn't tell me ahead of time, or they wrote duty limitations in a way that made it impossible for me to take that soldier to the field."

Army providers were missing opportunities to *shape the recovery environment* actively by formally communicating the results of command-directed evaluations of soldiers' mental status or communicating the duty limitations to which a soldier would need to be subjected given the mental illness.[9] And even when formal communication did happen, prior to 2011 it was handled exclusively on paper.[10] That meant there was no direct interaction between commanders and providers, which limited the ability of providers to get a richer understanding of a patient's occupational environment and of commanders to be engaged in helping shape a soldier's environment for recovery beyond the clinic. It was clear that the Army had to improve all three learning processes at the patient-care level.

Learning at the Clinic Level

Specialist Johnson's story that begins this chapter illustrates in particular some of the limitations of a system in which there is little or no clinic-level learning about patients. In the Army, given that learning at the patient-care level was ad hoc and driven by individual providers, it was not surprising that clinic-level learning processes were also ad hoc. What little clinic-level learning was taking place was largely confined to performance improvement projects and peer reviews.

In the Army, performance improvement projects, a commonly used clinic-level learning mechanism, were one-off provider-driven initiatives where lessons learned did not often survive provider or clinic leader turnover. In other words, these performance improvement projects generated reports and academic papers that never translated into sustained changes within clinics.

Peer reviews were discipline-based, so clinic members rarely got the opportunity to learn from other disciplines. For example, there was no institutional mechanism by which psychiatrists could improve their own practice by discussing cases with licensed clinical social workers. And even the discipline-based peer reviews themselves were suspect. "Even our peer review practices are broken," explained a provider with whom we spoke. "We select the cases we want to review, and we have our fellow professionals [exclusively in our specific discipline] give us feedback. It's not something that is tracked other than to document it so that we can show the Joint Commission that we did it!"[11]

There was no real learning from the peer reviews that fed into systematic improvement in the care practices of the clinic as a whole. This lack of learning may not have mattered when clinics were organized as collections of individual provider practices and demand for care was low enough that soldiers would always see their providers. But as demand for care grew, case complexity became greater, and there were not enough providers to staff all the cases. The need for such learning grew by leaps and bounds.

What does it look like when clinical-level learning is robust? It is about creating shared situational awareness across all care team members in a clinic to improve clinic performance collectively. That begins with all the providers in a clinic having a common understanding of the common mental health conditions they are treating within the clinic, so any new or unique cases can be immediately identified. It also requires that providers have an understanding of the history and current status of at-risk patients for whom they may have to provide care in the absence of those patients' usual providers.

To meet the growing demand for mental health care, Army clinics had to be staffed with multidisciplinary care teams consisting of physicians or nurse practitioners, psychologists, social workers, case managers, and other staff. These teams were designed to include a broad spectrum of experience, expertise, and treatment ability. In this new staffing approach, all clinicians would practice at the top of their licenses, so physicians and nurse practitioners would mostly do medication management, while psychologists and social workers would carry out psychotherapy. This division of clinical care meant that more coordination was needed across the different specialties to make sure there was collective ownership of patient care. Having collective ownership would create a treatment safety net when the provider of choice was not able to see the patient and enable positive continuation of treatment. That is where Specialist Johnson had been failed.

Clinic-level learning increases the capacity to treat complex cases in ways that would not be possible with the skills of a single provider. It requires building "time and space" into the clinic schedule for daily, weekly, and monthly meetings that involve care team members having collegial conversations across disciplinary boundaries.[12] Such meetings may *focus* on care for a single patient, but ideally they are designed to promote team psychological safety—"a shared belief that the team is safe for interpersonal risk taking"[13]—so team members can learn from each other. Meetings like these, held on a regular basis, afford the opportunity for members of a care team to discuss challenges and successes in treating patients and share lessons learned. That, in turn, does two critically important things: it empowers team members to ask for help when they need it; and it regularizes providers sharing their perspectives without having to be asked explicitly for help. Creating psychological safety is particularly important in multidisciplinary teams because of the historical power differences between psychiatrists, psychologists, and licensed clinical social workers arising from different lengths of training and scope of practice. A social worker, for instance, may not be comfortable suggesting alternative treatment options to a psychiatrist unless doing so is established as the norm within the team. Very little of that was happening in Army mental health care clinics when Specialist Johnson walked into that behavioral health clinic in 2011.

Hospital-Level Learning

In late 2010, more than sixty soldiers—all from one Army installation that was dealing with the aftermath of the "surge" that sent additional soldiers to Iraq and Afghanistan—were being admitted to non-Army hospitals each month for inpatient mental health care. During the first few months of this, no one really noticed—the surge was producing high numbers of soldiers in need. Eventually, though, it began to become a bit baffling.

Later, we walked through the admissions process that was generating these numbers. A soldier would present at the emergency department with a mental health "crisis" and be evaluated by emergency physician who was not a behavioral health provider. These physicians were routinely determining that more intensive psychiatric care was needed and would hand off the case to an emergency department nurse to transfer the patient to the inpatient ward. The nurse would call the hospital's psychiatric ward and ask whether a bed was available.

The hospital had twelve beds in its inpatient psychiatric ward, which had always been considered more than enough for the post's needs.

If no bed was available at the Army hospital, the soldier would automatically be sent for admission to a hospital in the surrounding community with an available psychiatric bed. Keep in mind that up to this point no behavioral health care provider at the Army hospital has seen the soldier in "crisis." And these soldiers at the civilian hospital would often keep the soldier for up to two weeks, whereas on the post the average stay was four days.

The bottom line was that soldiers who did not really need to be admitted were getting beds on and off the post because emergency physicians wanted to make sure they got care. For months and months, no one stopped to ask what might seem like obvious questions: Why are these numbers still so high? Are we doing something wrong? Do all these soldiers need inpatient care? Why are the soldiers admitted off post staying hospitalized for so long? Is the civilian hospital out to make money by keeping them?

Every hospital has some form of hospital-level learning that helps care teams develop and modify processes rapidly based on local needs, but these needs-solution pairs do not always systematically capture underlying technical or process problems or errors.[14] Hospital-level learning should enable identification and analysis of organizational errors across the hospital and provide the support needed to enable deliberate experimentation to address those errors.[15]

In the Army as a whole, there was limited focus on clinical or workflow errors related to mental health care. One could make a convincing case that there were very few rules or procedures in place beyond maximizing clinician productivity, maintaining access to care, and ensuring patient safety. The urgency of dealing with the increased mental health care needs resulting from the surge in Iraq and Afghanistan further masked such errors because leaders could not see the increased number of inpatient psychiatric admissions as a potential system failure in a situation where many of those admissions were simply unnecessary.

Only after hospital-level learning activities focused on identifying errors, analyzing them, and then setting up a deliberate experiment did inappropriate admissions drop at that Army installation.[16] The experiment involved changing the workflow to have the emergency department nurse call the inpatient psychiatric service and have a clinician sent to the waiting room to evaluate a soldier who might need to be admitted for inpatient care. That simple workflow change resulted in a decrease in the number of inappropriate admissions. "Now when soldiers are admitted to inpatient care," the inpatient chief noted, "we have made an assessment that they need that level of clinical care. Command teams now know that when we admit someone off-post, they have been seen by an Army mental health provider, and we know when and why the soldier was admitted."

That kind of hospital-level learning activity needed to be standardized and implemented across the Army.

Health System Learning

We were shocked during a visit to one Army post. We watched a soldier walk into a room where he could access the telebehavioral health system. We then saw the provider responsible for conducting a mental health screening for that soldier enter a different room to have a videoconference with that same soldier. The screening was taking place virtually—despite that the patient and provider were within walking distance of each other in the same building. If that seems nothing short of stupid to you, it did to us, too. How did it happen?

As soldiers began to return from Iraq and Afghanistan in the late 2000s, Army leaders grew increasingly concerned that they weren't providing much-needed—and *required*—mental health screenings. One reason was the lack of sufficient capacity to execute in-person assessments. So, the Army created a new, specific policy: 30 percent of all soldiers returning from the wars would be screened using telebehavioral health, the Army's system for face-to-face videoconferencing between soldiers and mental health providers. At the same time, there was an implicit assumption that wherever possible, the screenings would be done in person.

The hospital we visited was doing a great job of meeting that 30-percent requirement, but keeping to such a strict number sometimes required using telebehavioral health even when it didn't make any real sense. In the Army culture, compliance was a key driver of such decisions, and there was no mechanism for feedback and change. So, a poorly written, but quite specific, health system policy continued to be followed at that installation until someone finally asked the senior leader responsible for the policy whether that was what he had wanted. When the senior leader expressed his unhappiness that compliance had been substituted for common sense, the people at the clinic and hospital level were not the only ones to share the blame.

The story illustrates a lack of learning at the Army health system level—which requires that policies and system designs be examined for efficiency and effectiveness. It also requires the ability to mobilize and transfer knowledge, which also wasn't happening in the Army prior to 2010. At that time, the Army surgeon general had subject-matter experts and specialty consultants to advise on specific mental health care knowledge domains such as psychiatry and psychology. But these consultants did not directly affect system design. Each Army hospital designed its own system of care, and knowledge was not mobilized and transferred throughout the Army.

After the Embedded Behavioral Health model, a best practice described in chapter 3 that was created and piloted at Fort Carson, this incapacity for knowledge mobilization and transfer became quite apparent. The pilot project moved clinicians out of the hospital into distributed clinics that were within walking distance of a soldier's workplace. It successfully increased access to care and reduced the number of nondeployable 4th Infantry Division soldiers. And yet, the Army had no process for taking that model and implementing it at other Army locations that also faced the problem of providing care to soldiers in combat units that deployed frequently.

Learning from the Health Care Environment

In 2010, the Army was struggling to deal with the problem of soldier suicidal behavior. The number of soldiers who died by suicide had more than tripled, from 45 in 2001 to 156 in 2010.[17] There was no Army standard either for screening or clinically managing soldiers with suicidal behaviors. Providers relied on their own academic training or local best practices to identify and manage this high-risk population.

The head of the intensive outpatient care program at Fort Carson was grappling with the need to treat the growing number of soldiers exhibiting suicidal behaviors on her own post. She had been studying the research evidence on the efficacy of dialectical behavior therapy (DBT), a treatment developed for borderline personality disorder, in reducing self-harm, suicide ideation, and substance abuse in adolescents and adults.[18] She worked with her behavioral health chief and hospital leadership to create a new program that used DBT in an intensive outpatient format, and her team manually collected patient outcome data to show that the approach was effective at reducing suicidal behavior in enrolled soldiers. It was an example of one provider finding something in the literature that worked and then creating a local program. And it was a good thing, too, because it was 2013 before the Army had a standard clinical practice guideline for screening and treating soldiers with suicidal behaviors

Any health care system's ability to learn from the broader health care environment within which it functions is a critical capability. This is no less true for the Army than for any other system. There must be systematic ways to take advantage of academic research and innovation, both of which happen relentlessly and at a rapid pace. In 2014 alone, the National Institute of Mental Health funded nearly two thousand research projects in neuroscience, basic research, translational research, and intervention research.[19] Treatments designed and tested as a part of such research have the potential to improve dramatically the effectiveness and efficiency of care delivery. But while individual health care providers may be constantly learning to maintain their licensure, the Army health care system had not developed the processes needed to identify, evaluate, pilot, and diffuse learning from external research.

On top of that, other health care systems and other military services such as the Navy and the Marine Corps were also innovating. It was imperative that the Army figure out how to capture all the information being generated by these efforts and learn from it, but the Army had no way of systematically identifying and selecting research and best practices suited to the Army. Even when best practices were identified, there was no way to implement them. This learning from the health care environment needed to be developed—because that's what a learning health system *must* do.

Fixing the Problems

The Army had a lot of work to do, and it set out to address learning at all five levels.

Patient-Care Level

At the patient-care level, the Army transformation has fundamentally altered the three processes described earlier in the chapter. For instance, with respect to enhancing providers' clinical skills, the Army built in learning processes to train providers in evidence-based practice treatments for common mental health conditions such as post-traumatic stress disorder.

"When I first became a clinic chief," observed one behavioral health chief, "I had no idea if my providers were actually trained to treat combat-related trauma or suicidality, for that matter. Some of my providers hadn't managed a suicidal patient since their graduate education. Just two weeks ago, we trained all of our providers in the Collaborative Assessment and Management of Suicidality, which gave all of them an evidence-based practice to manage a condition that we see frequently enough where I don't want to have variation."

Providers reflect on their practice using records of their interactions with patients. These clinical notes are captured in the Army's electronic medical record (EMR), which must be used by all Army health care providers (behavioral health and otherwise). Providers would gather objective data using paper-based screening instruments they had learned to use as graduate students. Some providers had a preference for the Beck's Depression Inventory (BDI), while others preferred the Patient Health Questionnaire with nine questions (PHQ-9). It should come as no surprise that this process of collecting objective data varied significantly from provider to provider. The paper-based process added to one that was already time consuming for everyone involved, and then the provider still had to enter the calculated score manually into the EMR. The EMR was cumbersome enough that there was no guarantee the gathered data would be entered, let alone be used for later reflection. So the Army created a standardized set of screening instruments that providers were encouraged to use, with automated charting capabilities that would enable learning.

The patient-engagement process was another challenge. It was ad hoc, visit specific, and did not create consistent learning—all made worse by incomplete notes by providers. Research has shown that patient expectancy of treatment effectiveness, provider expectancy of treatment effectiveness, and the quality of the therapeutic alliance predict patient engagement and clinical improvement.[20] The Army's system-level commitment to measurement-based care and the use of systemically collected patient-reported outcome data to monitor and improve patient care led to the development of the Behavioral Health Data Portal (BHDP), an automated system to collect and report patient data.[21] This system now provides a quantitative foundation for assessing patient engagement in care. More important, it enables systematic learning in every patient visit. As a provider recently told us, "I now pull up BHDP in every patient visit. I can show the patient exactly where they are in this visit as compared to where they were three sessions ago. Even in the cases where the total score on the PTSD Checklist was the same, I can focus on specific areas such as sleep quality to keep the patient engaged."

Even though most Army providers are trained to use a biopsychosocial model for treating patients, providers often relied solely on patient input.[22] Even when they had approval to speak with family members and commanders, providers could not easily reach out to gather additional information. When we asked providers about why they did not talk to commanders to get additional context about a soldier, we heard a lot of explanations. "The soldier does not know exactly who his command team is," one provider said. "I have called the command team multiple times," another provider told us, "but they won't get back to me." Now that has been fixed.

The processes for *shaping recovery* begin with creating time in provider work schedules to engage commanders actively. Providers are now responsible for providing care for the seven hundred soldiers that would be in a typical army battalion. As a result, their patient panel consists mostly of soldiers from that battalion rather than all twenty thousand soldiers at a typical Army installation. The military is unique in that providers must share duty limitations with commanders. When a provider only has to take care of soldiers from a battalion, the provider also only has to work with six company commanders (the first leaders that have access to HIPAA-protected information for operational reasons) as opposed to all 120 company commanders on a post. That makes things like just having the right phone numbers for commanders, who change every two years, manageable.

Creating an electronic system for reporting duty limitations helped make communication between commanders and providers happen more quickly. Providers are now trained to write culturally competent duty limitations. As one commander told us, "Tell me what my soldier *can* do, not what they cannot do. That way, I can keep soldiers doing work that will keep them a part of the unit, and at the same time not hurt their recovery."

Clinic Level

At the clinic level, the learning processes focus on establishing shared team ownership of a patient's care and improving clinical workflows. The new system of care assigns responsibility for a soldier's care to the multidisciplinary team that staffs a clinic. The team creates shared ownership of a patients care through *morning huddles* and *multidisciplinary treatment planning meetings*. Each morning, the entire team comes together to identify any high-risk patients who may have been recently discharged from the hospital, any evaluated in an emergency department the previous night, or any that a provider is concerned about and wants the team to be aware of.

At a recent morning huddle in one of the Embedded Behavioral Health teams at Fort Riley, the nurse case manager went through the list of six patients who would be walking in that day for a safety check, including two who had been evaluated for a psychiatric crisis in the emergency department the night before. As they were wrapping up the meeting, one of the psychologists chimed in. "I'm worried about one of my soldiers I saw yesterday. He just broke up with his girlfriend and is having a tough time with his leadership. You all know that corporal's case. We've talked about him before." Most members of the team nodded in recognition.

Conversations like these are critical for a designated walk-in provider to go beyond a safety assessment and build on the care another team member has already provided. Such a conversation wouldn't have even been possible in the Army of 2010, but now they routinely happen throughout the Army's clinics.

Another new gathering, the multidisciplinary treatment planning (MDTP) meeting, expands a team's reach to include primary care providers, substance use care providers, and family advocacy care providers who may also be providing additional services. The MTDP allows members of the extended care team to share their individual clinical assessments so that the treatment plan each individual provider develops is aligned to common treatment goals. For example, the provider delivering psychotherapy for PTSD, the psychiatrist managing a soldier's medications, and the primary care provider helping that soldier address weight issues can work together to create a common treatment plan. The care team can also communicate with one voice to a soldier's commander that his weight gain is a side effect of treatment and offer clear duty limitations that support recovery.

The MDTP meetings also create the psychological safety for providers to ask for help in formulating a treatment plan. We observed an MDTP meeting and caught a good example how they draw on an entire team's expertise. "This soldier has some really complex issues related to sex," a provider told the group, "and I'm not equipped to deal with it. You've dealt with patients like this before," he said, turning to another provider on the team. "What should I do?" What might seem to be a routine question actually was a moment that highlighted the psychological safety that had been achieved within the team. The questioner was a psychiatrist who was turning to a licensed clinical social worker for help.

Also to facilitate learning at the clinic level, the Army has developed decision support tools that report clinical efficiency and effectiveness. These tools, discussed in greater detail in subsequent chapters, allow the clinic chief to use actual workload and outcome data to improve overall clinic performance.

Hospital Level

When it came to the Army-wide lack of hospital-level learning, the Army had to address a host of organizational, technical, and social barriers, beginning with the fact that no one was responsible for learning at the hospital level. The Army combined what had been three separate departments into a single, integrated Department of Behavioral Health, and made the head of Behavioral Health (BH) for each hospital responsible for the performance of all behavioral health clinics on a post. The Army also refined the digital infrastructure to accurately capture care delivered, and it created decision support tools that enable the behavioral health chief to look at an entire hospital and identify and analyze errors related to mental health services.

Several structured learning activities were instituted at the hospital level, including daily leader huddles (similar to those of the clinical teams) and monthly performance management sessions.

The daily leader huddle is a conference call chaired by the BH chief that involves all the clinic chiefs, after the latters' own morning huddles. It's a time for identifying near-term problems such as moving personnel to meet emergent or unanticipated demands, such as a provider having to take an emergency leave, or needing additional providers to screen soldiers returning from deployments to Iraq or Afghanistan.

The monthly performance management meetings allow the behavioral health chief to discuss operational issues that go beyond clinical efficiency to encompass clinical effectiveness. For instance, there's the issue of case notes. Providers are allowed to complete their case notes within seventy-two hours of a patient visit, but behavioral health chiefs prefer to have the notes completed the same day because a provider's recollection tends to diminish over time.

At one monthly meeting, a BH chief turned to one of his clinic chiefs and asked, "Why is your team so behind on notes? You have some providers that are barely making even their seventy-two–hour window!" "It's the same issue I've been bringing up in the morning huddles," the clinical chief responded. "For some reason, the AHLTA [the electronic medical record system] goes down every Tuesday, and the remote log-in system doesn't work well. Even if my providers wanted to, they couldn't complete the notes." The BH chief was able to take up the issue—one that would not have surfaced so quickly without the routine huddle—immediately afterward with the hospital's IT support team to ensure that updates that were causing outages were rescheduled for weekends rather than during the clinic's regular weekday hours.

Health System Level

Health system learning focuses on ensuring the effectiveness of system policies and enabling the diffusion of clinical and operational best practices from one hospital to others. A standard system design had to be developed and implemented to create a consistent patient experience of care across the network of thirty-four Army hospitals. Such a standard design could not be developed, implemented, and assessed to determine whether it was working and what changes might be needed, without a central team in Army headquarters organization responsible for managing mental health care across the entire Army.

A newly constituted central team designed the Army's standardized system of care using communities of practice that identified best practices in specific clinical microsystems that were proven to improve patient outcomes. Once these best practices were identified, the communities of practice codified the expected system behavior using policy documents, implementation handbooks, and performance standards. They also trained leaders to manage specific clinical microsystems, educated providers in new ways of working, and held monthly review sessions to support implementation efforts by sharing lessons from other implementation efforts across the Army.

The Army transitioned the system design communities of practice into program offices responsible for assessing the effectiveness of system policies and ensuring that implementation complied with the prescribed standards. The standardized system of care changed the flow of patients within military treatment facilities significantly, modified providers' workflows, and set new expectations of specific clinical skills. In short, it required new ways of working. There was a "knowing-doing gap"—knowing what works, and applying it in practice—that needed to be bridged.[23]

Consider the role of the Embedded Behavioral Health (EBH) program office in enabling Army-wide learning. The Army had issued a policy that required the implementation of an Embedded Behavioral Health clinic for each brigade combat team in the Army. The EBH program office published an implementation manual that guided individual hospitals through a structured process that covered staffing, infrastructure requirements, and metrics that would be used to assess implementation progress. The EBH program office had a monthly phone call involving five or six hospitals at a time, during which the program office would share its assessment of the EBH implementation at each hospital, using centralized data on system performance. Each hospital had an opportunity to share its own assessment based on its local data.

These two assessments did not always agree. For instance, staffing was a typical topic discussion in the early stages. The program office would highlight that EBH clinics were not staffed to the standard, and the hospitals would argue the opposite. Both were basing their arguments on data; the discrepancy stemmed from the data systems not accurately reflecting the actual clinics to which providers were assigned. Such issues could be addressed during the meeting and corrective action, such as updating provider assignments, could be taken immediately after.

Learning from the Health Care Environment

Best practices from other health care organizations are a valuable source of learning. The program offices for the standard clinical microsystems were given responsibility for identifying and incorporating best practices from other organizations. That's what Dr. Michael Faran, the Army's program director for Child and Family Behavioral Health, did.

A report by the Defense Health Board on pediatric care had found that mental health conditions were driving outpatient use for children and adolescents, and yet the system of care for that population was not very well defined in the Army in 2010.[24] Dr. Faran was looking for ways to improve the care for that vulnerable population when he met with Dr. Mark Weist, a pioneer in delivering mental health care in school settings.[25] Dr. Weist had demonstrated the power of moving care to "where it was needed" in the Baltimore City Public School System.[26] Dr. Faran wondered whether the same approach would work in the Army.

He ran a pilot program in Hawaii that moved social workers from the Army hospital to the Army-run schools, where the social workers could provide needed services on site. "We found that we were picking up a lot of kids that would never have been seen in a BH clinic," Dr. Faran observed, reflecting on the pilot project. "They were being identified by teachers and referred to the social worker in the school."

The pilot led to a decision to spread the idea across the Army, "branded" as School Behavioral Health. "In addition to meeting the known demand for services," Dr. Faran explained, "School Behavioral Health makes sense because it catches the unmet need—the children that never make it to a clinic. It uses a public health model that health care is moving towards, in that it identifies need early, engages key members of the community—parents and teachers—in enabling recovery, and encourages the use of evidence-based practices for treatment. An unintended consequence is that it also improves things like the climate and culture of the school."[27] Today, the Army has implemented School Behavioral Health in seventy-six schools, enhancing access to care to a known vulnerable population.

The Behavioral Health Service Line constantly scans for best practices in the larger civilian community. Army leaders collaborate with other large systems such as the Veterans Health Administration, Intermountain Health, and the Mayo Clinic to share best practices. The Army also identifies promising research in academia that is funded directly by the Department of Defense through the Medical Research and Material Command, as well as other federal- and foundation-supported research through participation in academic consortia such as the Military Suicide Research Consortium. Providers are encouraged to participate in their major professional conferences and, when they learn of best practices, notify the service line.

Lessons for Other Health Systems

The Army's learning architecture, shown in figure 4.1, illustrates the interplay within and across the five levels of learning. Health systems will benefit from developing a similar mapping of their own learning processes to transition to a learning mental health care system.

Provider-level learning is the core of any learning health care system. It occurs as providers enhance clinical skills, engage patients in care, and shape recovery through appropriate interactions with family members and employers. These learning activities have been essential for the Army's success in building a learning mental health system.

Clinically skilled providers are the building blocks of organizational learning. They must sustain clinical skills to maintain their independent licensure. Yet, not every independently licensed provider has the skills needed to meet the care needs of a health system's beneficiary population. Once a health system maps out needed clinical competencies (based on known and projected service needs), it can either train its providers, as the Army did in training its providers in evidence-based PTSD treatments, or hire new providers with those competencies.

Mapping the processes used to collect patient-reported outcome data and understanding how the collected data are used in the treatment planning process provide an initial assessment of patient engagement activities. Measurement-based care has the potential to increase patient engagement and reduce treatment dropout. Many health systems use a time-consuming manual process for collecting objective data that relies on paper instruments and hand scoring and reduces the actual time available to spend with the patient. Furthermore, not having longitudinal data may negatively affect treatment planning. The Army's approach of automating data collection and standardizing reporting makes it easier for providers to incorporate the data into treatment planning, which in turn translates to improved patient engagement and clinical care.

As mentioned earlier, the Army is unique because providers are required to engage a soldier's "employer"—commanders—to shape the recovery environment. Given the limited ability for a mental health care system to shape occupational environments in civilian settings, those systems must create venues for actively engaging family members in treatment to enable recovery.

Other systems should also consider the Army's practice of selecting the best leader for the role of clinic chief, as opposed to the most qualified clinician.

As health systems begin to integrate mental health care into overall medical care, they must address the hospital-level coordination issues that emerge from synchronizing different practices. They need to develop organization rules and procedures that are not only consistent across different mental health clinics, but also consistent with other medical care. Mental health providers may not be comfortable documenting in a shared medical record. One of the early challenges in integrating substance use clinical care in the Army was the unwillingness of providers to document anything more than "Patient seen, patient not a risk to harm self or others, see paper record" in the electronic medical record. If the only analysis of the workflow was to determine whether there was some documentation in the medical record, it would have completely missed the fact that the documentation itself was not particularly helpful.

The Army experience shows the importance of having a behavioral health chief at the hospital level to manage mental health care. She needs to understand how the hospital works, because she will depend on the hospital for critical activities such as provider credentialing and privileging. There are also social barriers that need to be overcome if the behavioral health chief is not a physician. One BH chief, a clinical psychologist, recalled to us her first experience in a meeting of hospital leaders. "I

TABLE 4.1 Questions to help enable learning

LEARNING LEVEL	QUESTION
Patient care	Do providers have the clinical skills required to meet patient needs?
	Do providers engage their patients in care?
	Do providers engage family members and employers to shape recovery?
Clinic	Does the care team own a patient's care?
	How can the team improve its work practices?
Hospital	Can the hospital identify and analyze clinical and workflow errors?
	Does the hospital enable deliberate experimentation?
	Can the hospital diffuse learning to its constituent clinics?
Health system	Can the health system assess the effectiveness of system policies?
	Can the health system mobilize knowledge from one hospital to the next?
Environment	Can the health system identify external knowledge it can use?

walked into the meeting, and the hospital commander said, 'Thank you all for coming.' He introduced me by name, told the group I was the new behavioral health chief, and said, 'She's not really a doctor, but we won't hold it against her.'"

Hospital-level learning activities such as leader huddles make it easier to solve immediate resource and infrastructure problems. The monthly performance management meetings identify problem areas that can be addressed either though change in system design or, in some cases, refining a policy.

In a rapidly changing health care environment, health systems have to enhance their absorptive capacity—their ability to adapt or make changes to established work practices seamlessly—so they can translate relevant research into practice and pull in best practices from other organizations. The Army had to grow its absorptive capacity through the continual engagement of its program with the thirty-four Army hospitals that were implementing the standard system of care. Other health systems would benefit from assessing their own absorptive capacities by examining whether they have been able to incorporate changes from outside their organizations.

As for the Army, benchmark data are also gathered from peer health systems such as the VA, the Israeli Defense Forces, and the British Army for assessing performance and identifying best practices that can be adapted.

The five levels of learning discussed in this chapter provide a framework that can be used by other health systems to examine their own learning processes. Table 4.1 summarizes the kinds of questions systems should ask to determine where their own learning stands, and what they need to do to enable further learning.

Chapter 5

BUILDING ANALYTICS CAPABILITIES TO SUPPORT DECISION MAKING

In April 2011, Lieutenant General Eric Schoomaker—then the Army surgeon general—was called to testify before the US Senate Committee on Appropriations in a hearing on Department of Defense health programs for the coming fiscal year. One of the committee members, Senator Barbara Mikulski of Maryland, asked him whether the Army had an adequate number of mental health professionals to provide the services soldiers and their families needed.

"I think the Nation is facing a problem with mental health professionals—," Lieutenant General Schoomaker began to reply, but Senator Mikulski cut him off.

"No," she said. "Do you have it? I am not talking about the Nation."

Lieutenant General Schoomaker continued in the same direction. "As a microcosm of the Nation, we have problems, especially as—"

And again Senator Mikulski interrupted him. "Again, I am not being—I really—"

Finally, Lieutenant General Schoomaker got to the point. "We have problems, ma'am."[1]

It was a stunning exchange. Several years into a crisis created by a lack of available mental health care in the Army, a senator asked whether the Army had enough providers, and the Army surgeon general could not answer. He, like everyone else within the Army health care system, did not have the data. The Army, like the rest of the Department of Defense, did not know how many providers it required to meet the needs of its soldiers and other beneficiaries. Why couldn't these questions be answered?

The health care digital infrastructure—all the health information technology the Army was using—was fragmented, difficult to integrate, and limited in scope. It frequently produced information that was applicable only to a single Army post. That information was riddled with errors due to mistakes in personnel files and other data uploaded manually by administrative staff in each hospital. It didn't include any information on the clinical outcome of the care itself. As a result, it couldn't be used to answer critically important questions: Where is the care provided? How effective is that care? How efficiently do clinics provide it?

The Army had a large amount of data and information, but struggled to leverage it systematically to improve care quality and patient outcomes (see table 5.1). In the end, it left Army leaders uninformed about how many more providers they needed to meet soldiers' demand for care—and thus unable to respond to members of Congress.

TABLE 5.1 Army health care digital infrastructure

DIGITAL INFRASTRUCTURE COMPONENTS	DESCRIPTION AND ISSUES
Defense Enrollment Eligibility-Reporting System (DEERS)	Captures demographic, occupational, and contact data of all soldiers and other beneficiaries eligible for care. The data in this system were trustable and consistently validated.
Defense Medical Human Resources System-internet (DMHRSi)	Captures human resources data on manpower, personnel, labor cost, education, and training from a variety of sources. Data in this system were not always trustable, because the system relied on each provider to enter data manually every two weeks.
Medical Expense and Performance Reporting System (MEPRS)	Captures manpower, cost distribution, and expense data at the work-center level. Data in this system were not trustable because work centers were defined differently by each hospital.
Composite Health Care System (CHCS)	Captures patient registration data, appointment scheduling, and tracking at a given military treatment facility. Data were not trustable because each hospital defined its own appointment types and provider templates.
Armed Forces Health Longitudinal Technology Application (AHLTA)	Captures outpatient medical records. A single record is created for a patient at a given hospital and is regularly updated with encounter notes at a given hospital. The data were not usable for automatically analyzing patient-level or population-level outcomes.
Essentris	Captures inpatient medical records for a given hospital. Unlike AHLTA, a new patient record is created each time the patient is admitted to the hospital. The data captured in Essentris were not usable for automatically analyzing patient-level or population-level outcomes.

Analytics, the systematic application of mathematics and computer science techniques to find meaningful patterns in data, is now being employed to enable better decision making in the delivery and management of mental health care services. Prior to 2012, Army hospitals conducted their own analytics because so little was performed at the system level and made available to local facilities. The Behavioral Health Service Line (BHSL) led an extensive process to correct errors in the source data, making the information more reliable at the system level. It then developed tools that integrated the Army's information technology systems to answer three key questions: How well are we using our existing providers (clinician productivity assessment)? How many providers do we need (prescriptive capacity planning)? Is the care provided effective (clinical care effectiveness)? These tools form the basis of the digital infrastructure that today supports the Army's learning behavioral health system.

Clinician Productivity Assessment

A clinician's time is the most valuable resource in any mental health care system. In most health care systems, providers are to some extent motivated to use their time in the clinic to conduct as many appointments as possible because they are paid only for those they perform. In the Army's health care system, like most governmental organizations, providers are paid according to a set salary, as long as they perform enough appointments to reach a minimum standard. That standard is usually expressed by the number of RVUs that are "produced" by those appointments and is, therefore, called a "productivity standard." In systems such as the Army's, someone in a leadership position sets a productivity standard and providers receive their full salary (including bonuses) if they reach it.

Before the Army vastly expanded its behavioral health clinics amid the sharp increase in demand resulting from the wars in Iraq and Afghanistan, it used a single productivity standard for each type of provider working in any Army clinic. However, as the demand for behavioral health care skyrocketed and the Army opened numerous types of new clinics—which called for its providers to perform different numbers and types of appointments—the single productivity standard became a huge problem. Some providers could meet the standard, but others who were asked to perform tasks that didn't produce RVUs, such as working with commanders to provide better support for their soldiers with mental health problems, could not. Providers felt the Army's productivity standards did not reflect the full scope of work they were being asked to do. And those providers were absolutely correct.

The Army's new standard system of care was the first step in fixing the issue. As the Army established standard clinical programs throughout all its hospitals, it was able to set corresponding workload standards that made sense for providers. The revised productivity standards published in 2013 for the new system of care provided a level of granularity that had not existed before to the nature of work done by different types of providers. For example, the productivity requirements for a psychiatrist (detailed in table 5.2) were specified based on the amount of clinical care that must be provided in the clinic where the psychiatrist worked. The standards were expressed in the expected RVU production for a day, a month, and a year.

Developing workload standards consistent with the work providers were asked to do was a major step forward, but the fragmentation of the Army's digital infrastructure made it difficult for providers' leaders at the local level to view how their production measured up against the Army's standard. Prior to 2011, many hospital leaders developed their own homegrown solutions. At one location, the behavioral health chief shared a complex spreadsheet that he had created for tracking provider productivity. This chief had listed all sixty-five providers by the type of clinic. He then manually entered the total appointments they had scheduled (new patients, established patients, group therapy, walk-ins, others), the patients that did not show up for the appointments, the appointments cancelled by the hospital, and the RVUs produced. This labor-intensive, manual-entry monthly process had allowed him to develop his own eponymous efficiency index that showed him how well he was using his providers.

Other Army hospitals did not have the same spreadsheet, nor did they try to develop their own version of the spreadsheet. Some of the behavioral health chiefs were so busy just trying to take care of soldiers that showed up at their clinics. They didn't have time to drill any deeper than to make sure that their providers were meeting their RVU targets.

There had to be an easier way to integrate these data systematically and provide them in a usable fashion for leaders and providers. That came with the establishment of an analytics capacity within the Army's service-level leadership team, which gave the Army the centralized capability to calculate and display its providers' productivity in all its hospitals. That effort began with a painstaking process to realign the administrative codes so they reflected the new, standard clinics being established by Army hospitals. The newly organized data were then combined into a single tool called the Capacity Analysis and Reporting Tool (CART).

CART is a spreadsheet-based analytics tool updated monthly by the Behavioral Health Service Line analytics team for the use of providers, administrators, and leaders at all levels. Its workbook format makes the data and the analysis transparent and traceable to the user. Two of CART's strengths as an analytic tool are its ease of distribution as an Excel workbook and its feature that allows leaders to

TABLE 5.2 Example of revised provider productivity standards in 2013

PROVIDER SPECIALTY	CLINIC / MISSION ROLE	12-MONTH ROLLING TARGET (eRVUs)	12-MONTH ROLLING MINIMUM THRESHOLD	WEEKLY HOUR EQUIVALENT IN CLINIC	"TYPICAL DAY" (ADJUSTED FOR AVAILABILITY) eRVU TARGET EQUIVALENT	21 CLINIC DAY MONTH EQUIVALENT
Psychiatrist	Single or multispecialty BH clinic	3,300	2,475	30.0	16.9	355.4
	Telebehavioral health hub	3,069	2,302	30.0	15.7	330.5
	BH provider in primary care clinic (IBHC/PC)	3,300	2,475	30.0	16.9	355.4
	School-based BH program	3,300	2,475	30.0	16.9	355.4
	Child-focused mission (CAFBHS, child and adolescent clinics)	2,860	2,145	30.0	14.7	308.0
	Integrated pain management clinic	3,300	2,475	30.0	16.9	355.4
	TBI	3,300	2,475	30.0	16.9	355.4
	GME / trainee faculty	2,200	1,650	20.0	11.3	236.9
	Embedded Behavioral Health (EBH)	3,300	2,475	30.0	16.9	355.4
	Department chief (admin)	440	330	4.0	2.3	47.4
	Subordinate chiefs	2,200	1,650	20.0	11.3	236.9

carry out point-and-click analysis. CART also provides indicators of potential data integrity challenges. For example, the assessment of capacity by availability of providers to create health care value begins with accurate personnel data. Care that cannot be tied directly to a provider reporting clinical time in the personnel management system is summarized in the "workload without manpower" metric and indicates a data-quality issue local leaders can easily investigate.

At first, though, most chiefs of behavioral health departments vigorously resisted CART, which they saw as a tool that contained inaccurate information and wouldn't help them manage their clinics. As one chief said, "I spend more time fighting with the service line about [the data in] CART than managing my own people!" But when the service line team looked into complaints, they usually found errors in the source data, not problems with the tool itself. Even Fort Carson, where one of the present authors served as the behavioral health chief, had errors in its personnel files. One psychiatrist was incorrectly classified as a family physician. A psychologist who had completed training and was independently licensed to practice was labeled as a trainee, and so received no RVUs for the care he provided. Once the behavioral health chiefs corrected the errors in the source data being inputted by their staffs, the inaccuracies in the CART disappeared, as did their resistance to using the tool to manage their clinical teams' productivity.

As the department chiefs became more comfortable with the accuracy of CART, they began to apply its features within their management practices. Learning accelerated as a result. At a glance, they could determine whether a provider was not meeting the expected productivity standard. They could also benchmark the performance against other providers in the clinic, hospital, region, or Army as a whole.

Department chiefs also used the CART to solve problems in unexpected ways. One department chief discussed how he used CART to address a significant staff morale problem among his social workers. "They were right," he told us, smiling. "The CART data show they are providing a majority of the psychotherapy, but their salary is maxed out. I don't have the funds to give them financial bonuses, so instead I give them half-days off or allow them to work four ten-hour days. They are still meeting all their productivity standards and they know the Army appreciates them."

CART was the culmination of a multiyear effort to establish productivity standards that made sense to clinicians and leaders at all levels, correct errors in source data, and bring those data together into a single, easily viewable tool. With CART in hand, the Army could begin to examine more complex issues that were standing in the way of building a learning behavioral health system.

Centralized Capacity Planning

As the testimony before the Senate that opened this chapter illustrates, the Army faced serious challenges when it came to estimating accurately the number and mix of clinicians needed to support the changing demand for mental health care, which is also known as capacity planning. The Army's capacity planning process before 2013 was an annual hospital-specific process in which the local leaders would make guesstimates of their needed care capacity based on the prior year's workload and a gut sense of potential growth. These leaders were carrying out their "analyses" with low-quality, incomplete information. In addition, because approximately 30 percent of the beneficiaries on each Army post move from one location to another each year, leadership at a given Army hospital had no real sense of the needs of the soldiers and family members that would seek care in their facility in the following year.

Capacity planning is important because it determines how many clinical staff a hospital tries to hire and maintain on staff. If an Army hospital underestimates its need for providers, the impact on beneficiaries is significant because they may have to seek care in the local community. Given that a large number of Army posts are located within health professional shortage areas (HPSAs) for mental health care, inaccurate estimates of capacity translate into patients waiting in long lines to see someone from among the already insufficient number of community providers.[2]

Another consequence of hospitals underestimating the clinical capacity they need is the pressure placed on its clinical staff, which often leads to burnout. Providers interviewed by the MIT team in 2012 showed all three dimensions of burnout: they said they were exhausted; they felt frustrated that the system seemed focused on paying for volume rather than care quality; and, worst of all, they felt they were not effective in helping their patients or clients.[3]

The capacity planning model in use at the time, called the Army's Automated Staffing Assessment Model (ASAM), significantly underestimated the work providers actually performed and failed to capture all the administrative tasks providers in the military health system were required to perform. Once the Army developed its productivity assessment tool (CART), it better understood how busy its providers really were and could then build a tool that determined how many more it needed to meet its beneficiaries' mental health needs. It came up with a hybrid capacity planning approach that incorporated known population health needs as well as a demand-based adjustment based on operational tempo. This new design allowed for more precise estimates of nonclinical provider workload, the major problem with the ASAM tool. The new Distribution Matrix Tool (DMT) was released in 2014.[4]

The DMT uses the productivity standards to detail the number of clinical staff each hospital needs in each of its behavioral health clinics. This new mission-based workload specification for each core provider type, combined with a multidisciplinary team structure, serves as the foundation for building a patient-centered care team. System-level staff reassess capacity annually and work with the resource management teams to ensure that funds are available for each hospital to hire the staff it needs, according to the DMT. Two limitations still remain, even with this model: the Army posts continue to provide their population needs projections, and the model does not capture demand variation due to deployments. The first limitation is mitigated to some extent by assessing at the third quarter of each year, when most permanent change of stations would have been completed.

Clinical Care Effectiveness

There were two technical gaps the Army had to fill to answer the question of whether the care it provided was effective. The first was to develop a method to perform measurement-based care and, therefore, generate data on clinical outcomes (which are explained below). The second was to make the clinical outcome data interpretable for groups of patients over time by defining something called an "episode of care." The Army realized that if it could solve these two problems and create a consistent flow of information on the effectiveness of the care its providers were delivering, it would open unprecedented opportunities to learn.

Measurement-Based Care

Measurement-based care (MBC)—the systematic administration of symptom rating scales and use of the results to drive clinical decision making at the level of the individual patient—has been shown to improve the efficacy of mental health care by many in the field.[5] That's a clear indication that MBC helps providers learn about the care they're providing to their patients and use that information to improve their treatment. Unfortunately, few health care systems have implemented MBC and even fewer have developed ways to use the information it produces, also called clinical outcome data, to improve how their clinics provide care. Most systems instead rely on measures of structure such as how many providers are trained in evidence-based practices, and measures of process such as how frequently therapy is provided, as substitutes for a measure of whether a patient's symptoms have improved with treatment.

The Army developed the Behavioral Health Data Portal (BHDP) to solve this problem and implement measurement-based care in all its clinics. While in the waiting room before an appointment, patients digitally complete—through BHDP—standard instruments that quantify their symptoms. Through a secure web-based interface, BHDP presents the data to the patient's provider prior to the start of the appointment, giving her a structured view of the symptoms that have improved and those that have not. The provider sees the data from that day's appointment on a graph that includes the patient's responses prior to past appointments, which gives her a clear depiction of how the patient's symptoms have changed throughout the course of treatment.

After a multiyear development and dissemination process, all Army outpatient clinics now use BHDP with their adult patients. As of the end of 2017, BHDP was used in more than 834,000 appointments per year, which is greater than 70 percent of all appointments.[6] In total, patients have submitted information through BHD in conjunction with more than four million outpatient appointments—a powerful foundation of data that supports learning on all levels. But the usefulness of those data would be severely limited if the Army couldn't organize them into a simple and meaningful format that describes the impact of the treatment it provides to its patients.

Episode of Care

An episode of care is a "series of health-related events with a beginning, an end, and a course, all related to a particular health problem that exists continuously for a delimited period of time."[7] Episodes of care are hard to define because health care is complex, often involving multiple clinical teams.[8] There are few guidelines for defining episodes of care, and because patients often move in and out of regular contact with the health care system, the task of marking the start and end of an episode of care can seem arbitrary.[9]

Software for generating episodes of care, such as the INGENIX Symmetry's Episode Treatment Groups or the Thompson Reuters Medstat Medical Episode Grouper (MEG), are less-than-ideal solutions because they use proprietary algorithms that are not visible to users.[10] Since each software system has its own propriety approach for classifying episodes, the episode designations are not compatible.[11] The grouping algorithms in both software programs do not emulate practice patterns, and there is significant variation in cost within episodes and across episodes.[12] These three factors highlighted the need for the Army to develop its own easily understandable method for designating an episode of care for mental health conditions.

The Army partnered with the MIT team, under the direction of one of the present authors, to use the data it had recently corrected and reorganized. The team studied how Army providers used codes representing the initial diagnosis and subsequent treatment when documenting the care they provided. They used the information to set definitions for the beginning and end of an episode of care. Finally, the team applied the definition to the rapidly growing clinical outcome data being generated through BHDP. The result provided the Army with the ability to see how severe its patients' symptoms were at the beginning, middle, and end of treatment—a major step that enabled several advancements that would come soon after.

Lessons for Other Health Systems

In 2016 alone, global spending on health analytics reached $6.2 billion, and the market for health analytics tools is projected to reach nearly $14.9 billion by 2022.[13] Most of this spending was focused on traditional health care, not mental health care. The Army experience provides a road map for developing mental health care–specific analytics capabilities to answer questions about whether a health system has the right mix and number of providers, whether those providers are being used efficiently, and whether the care delivered is effective.

Many health systems have patchwork digital infrastructures for managerial accounting, personnel management, beneficiary enrollment, patient appointment scheduling, clinical care record keeping, and billing. The Army's approach of making sure data are trustable and accurately reflect patient flows can be replicated by other health care systems. When the digital infrastructure has trustable data, the digital imprint—what the data within different health information technology systems say about the delivery of mental health care—reflects how mental health care is organized and delivered. When the digital imprint and the lived experiences of patients and providers diverge, learning is severely limited.

The Army's mix of descriptive and prescriptive analytics tools are designed to support decision making at the health system, hospital, clinic, and provider levels of analysis. These tools use the same underlying data that have been verified and validated by both the hospital and the Army. Creating this single source of truth is a necessary step for building usable mental health analytics.

Health systems can build and use an Excel-based clinician productivity tool like the Army's CART so that providers can see their performance against peers at their hospital and across the health system. Clinic chiefs can also examine efficiency by examining the mix of disease and treatment approaches across their patient population to use their limited clinical assets in the best way.

The Army's prescriptive capacity planning tool combines known population health needs, the expected standard of care, and projected health needs to ensure that needed health care can be provided at the right time and at the right place. Such a tool would help other health systems plan for care for comorbid mental health care and chronic conditions.

The Army's episode of care framework is one of the few such tools that can be assessed and easily replicated by other health systems. It combines clinical and administrative data in a manner that allows providers to improve their clinical care and administrators to manage the practice. It is the very type of tool needed as health systems move to managing comorbid medical and mental health conditions.

Chapter 6

MANAGING PERFORMANCE IN A LEARNING BEHAVIORAL HEALTH SYSTEM

Lieutenant Colonel Johnson, chief of the Department of Psychiatry at a large Army hospital, gathered the clinical and administrative behavioral health leaders at the annual off-site meeting. Their agenda: review their performance in the prior year and set the strategic plan for the upcoming year. The Departments of Psychology and Social Work would meet separately and develop their own plans.

In the weeks before the off-site, the department administrator had combed through several administrative databases of information on how many appointments the psychiatrists had performed, the RVUs they had generated, the number of days patients had to wait for appointments, and how frequently they required admission to inpatient care. As was the usual process, he spent several days doing calculations by hand, closely adhering to the minimum standards and goals Lieutenant Colonel Johnson had set the year before. A couple of days before the off-site, he provided Johnson with his results in the form of several bar graphs.

Lieutenant Colonel Johnson and the clinic chiefs spent much of the off-site meeting comparing the data with that from the year earlier. The department's performance had shown no improvement. Johnson wanted an explanation. And one after the other, the clinic chiefs blamed problems they saw in the data, which they believed made the performance of their respective teams look worse than it actually was.

"This RVU information is misleading," insisted one clinic chief. "I had a provider out of work on a medical leave for months." Relative value units, as we explained in chapter 3, are a measure hospitals use to compare the resources required to perform various clinical services. "I don't think these data even account for how the Psychology Department has affected my numbers," another clinic chief complained. "Those guys haven't pulled their weight when it comes to on-call responsibilities for more than a year, and time after time my psychiatrists end up having to leave the clinic. It's a serious drag on our productivity." A third chief described how the data couldn't possibly account for the reality of his clinic. "You all know our patients have symptoms that are way more severe than the rest of you," he said. "Those cases required so much more time from my providers." The one thing all the clinic chiefs agreed on was that their psychiatrists were working extremely hard and that every clinic needed more of them to be hired. They said that every year.

Lieutenant Colonel Johnson had heard all the complaints before. He was sure there was some truth to them, but it was almost impossible to know how much. The data he had in front of him certainly didn't help much. He had no confident sense of how efficient his clinics really were or how his teams performed compared to those in other, similar Army hospitals. He had no idea whether any of his peers, chiefs of other departments of psychiatry, had found ways to solve the administrative problems, such as expediting appointments for patients with the most severe diagnoses, that were dragging down his department's performance numbers.

Limited Amounts of Useful Data

Lieutenant Colonel Johnson's dilemma was typical in 2010. Behavioral health leaders at all levels of the Army had limited amounts of useful data with which to make decisions. To find those data, staff members had to dig into multiple databases. Hospitals generated their own reports when leaders wanted to examine performance. The Army didn't have a centrally maintained data platform that displayed common behavioral health metrics. There was no assurance that the methodology used to generate a report on some aspect of system performance—say, time between admissions—would be the same in any two Army hospitals. That made comparing performance against other hospitals nearly impossible.

The MIT team observed this very problem firsthand. At one Army installation, we saw staff correctly compute the *thirty-day readmission rate* for psychiatric hospitalizations using the discharge date as starting point. At another, we saw staff use the date of admission. When we asked about using the admission date as the starting point, staff justified their process: "In our purchased care data, the only date is the admissions date, so we used that." They were relying on billing data that needed to capture only the date of admission and the length of stay to determine cost of an inpatient admission. The staff could have easily computed the discharge date, but they neglected to do so.

This had ripple effects in terms of how that hospital assessed its own care quality. While it can be argued that a readmission within thirty days may not necessarily indicate poor care quality, it is seen as a useful tool for controlling the cost of care.[1] In using the date of admission to compute the readmission rate, that hospital was given a false sense of security that soldiers were not being readmitted frequently. The hospital that was doing it right had spent more time thinking about the problem, and it calculated the discharge date based on the admission and length of stay (which was available). Even though the numbers looked bad, the report helped leaders at that installation focus on the right areas to improve quality of care.

Neither the Army nor the military health system (MHS) as a whole had really thought through how to examine the performance of mental health care delivery. The MHS had recognized the need to develop a performance management system that would allow the Department of Defense to measure progress against the Quadruple Aim, which added readiness of the military to deploy to Iraq, Afghanistan, or elsewhere by extending the triple aims of improving the experience of care, improving population health, and reducing the per capita cost of health care.[2] The MHS adopted the balanced scorecard (BSC) approach, which had been successful in the Mayo clinic, to track progress toward the Quadruple Aim, adding "Learning and Growth" as the fifth area for tracking progress in a strategy map (figure 6.1).[3]

The MHS developed strategic imperatives, the critical activities that would help the MHS achieve one of more of the Quadruple Aims, but could not match strategic imperatives to performance measures and strategic initiatives for mental health care. For instance, a task force was set up to develop the metrics after psychological health and resiliency was defined as a strategic imperative. One of the

Learning and Growth			Per Capita Cost	Experience of Care				Population Health	Readiness	
Fully capable MHS workforce	Using research to improve performance	Effective knowledge management	Align incentives to promote outcomes and increase value for stakeholders	Personal relationships with your doctor	24/7 access to your medical home	Wounded warrior care	Evidence-based care	Engaging patients in healthy behaviors	Psychological health and resiliency	Individual and family medical readiness

FIGURE 6.1. Partial MHS strategy map in 2010. Adapted from the slide titled "What Value When?" in Middleton and Dinneen (2011).

present authors was a member of that task force. After two years of biweekly meetings, the group concluded that it did not have enough understanding of the structure, processes, and outcomes related to the provision of mental health care across the Army, Navy, Air Force, and Marine Corps to develop an MHS-wide mental health balanced scorecard.

The Army could not do it alone, either. Lieutenant General Eric Schoomaker, the Army surgeon general at that time, was a strong believer in the BSC approach, and in his guidance to commanders shortly after taking that assignment had written, "Use the BSC as a guide in all command and management functions with conscious disciplined application, it truly works!"[4] But while he and other Army leaders expected the Army's behavioral health system of care to contribute to achieving the Quadruple Aim, there was nothing in the Army's balanced scorecard on how that could be achieved for mental health care. There was no way for Army leadership to know which hospitals were excelling and which were struggling to achieve the Quadruple Aim. The Army did not have a digital infrastructure or analytics (as discussed in the previous chapter) that could be trusted, so it persisted with the management approach in which each Army hospital was responsible for developing its own metrics and managing its own performance.

Without a common set of metrics, opportunities to learn from peers in other Army hospitals was generally limited to annual conferences or ad hoc discussions. System-level leaders rarely learned which hospitals had the best practices that should be disseminated to other hospitals.

A Lack of System-Wide Standards

Sitting in his office the day after the off-site, Lieutenant Colonel Johnson found himself focusing on efficiency problems—the one thing that was very clear from the data he had seen. He wondered whether his providers were seeing enough patients each day, but he had no system-wide standard to turn to as a reference. The fact was that the Army allowed Johnson to set his own workload standards, as long as he could justify them to his hospital commander through the performance-based assessment model, the fiscal oversight process in use at the time, which allowed for plenty of subjective adjustment at the local level.

Lieutenant Colonel Johnson thought about whether he should try to convince the hospital commander to give him funds to hire more psychiatrists, or whether to require his psychiatrists to pack more appointments into their schedules. Nothing from the system level set a floor or ceiling on how many providers his department could hire. If he could persuade his hospital commander of the need, he could hire more. But that lack of standards—the complete absence of any guidance from the system level that estimated how many clinicians would be needed to meet the behavioral health needs of the patients enrolled to his hospital—weighed heavily on him. "I really have no way to know for sure whether we have enough providers," he thought to himself.

Then Lieutenant Colonel Johnson recalled a meeting he had had recently with the behavioral health staff member at the regional medical command (an intermediary headquarters between his hospital and the system-level leaders in the surgeon general's office). The regional behavioral health leader had made a new point of emphasis: "Ensuring that patients have sufficient access to care is the key to good care," he had said. Regional headquarters wanted all possible steps to be taken to expand access to behavioral health care.

"But the hospital commander, just last week, said the budget was out of control and said the entire hospital would hire only a few new providers this year," Lieutenant Colonel Johnson thought to himself, scratching his head at yet another instance of mixed messages from two different levels of leadership. Obviously, both access to care and fiscal responsibility were important priorities, but which was the higher priority? Johnson had no idea. He chuckled cynically to himself. "I'm sure they'll be a new top priority next month, anyway."

In 2010, the strategic-level priorities seemed to be inconsistent and evolving. Local leaders made decisions based almost completely on local factors and rarely to achieve a strategic goal set out at the system level. The Army's priorities seemed to change from month to month, from ensuring access to care to increasing provider efficiency as measured in RVUs to maximizing patient satisfaction with the experience of care. On and on the priorities changed. And while the successive surgeon generals published broad organizational goals each year in a balanced scorecard format, how they applied to behavioral health care was interpreted differently in each hospital.

Lieutenant Colonel Johnson did wonder, though, how effectively his providers delivered care. How frequently did their patients get better? He suspected, based on informal conversations he would have with soldiers and nonmedical leaders while making his usual visits through his clinics, that some cases were more successful than others. Why was that? How many of his providers used evidence-based practices and how many were using less-effective therapies? How many patients felt their psychiatrists were working well with them? The Psychiatry Department chief found it so frustrating that there were no data available to help him answer those questions.

He wasn't the only one lacking data. Leaders at the system level had little to help them assess how each hospital was performing in any area beyond basic administrative functions. They received no direct information about the effectiveness of behavioral health care. Even if they could see that Dr. Thomas, a psychiatrist at one hospital, seemed to be "perfect"—completing ten patient appointments per day, finishing his notes on time, coding them properly in the electronic health record, and keeping up to date on all required training—they had no idea whether the care he provided was effective. Did the patients that came to his clinic have significantly fewer symptoms of depression or PTSD after treatment, or not? The system offered no way to tell. From the system level all the way down to Lieutenant Colonel Johnson, leaders simply did not know how many patients that were under the care of their providers actually got better and how many perhaps even got worse.

In 2010, the situation was nearing a tipping point. Pressure from members of Congress and very senior Army leaders grew steadily. They demanded to know how much progress the Army Medical Command was making in the fight against mental illness among soldiers and their family members. How were medical leaders identifying the most effective clinical strategies and replicating them across the Army? What gaps still existed? When would they be filled?

A performance management system could help answer those questions. For the first time ever, the Army medical system began to put in place the key pieces to create one.

Creating the Context for Performance Management

Prior to 2012, the Army could not have built a performance management system capable of providing what was needed because the Army lacked three critical pieces that had to be in place for it to work: reliable, meaningful data; a clear, coherent leadership organization for overall behavioral health care; and leaders at the local level. Let's look at each of these in turn.

First, such a system required reliable data on all aspects of how behavioral health care was delivered at the local level. As the previous chapter describes, those data would need to provide insight into several important aspects of behavioral health care delivery, including how the clinical staff was structured and organized, how efficiently clinics were running, how closely providers adhered to evidence-based practices, how frequently patients' symptoms were resolved, and indicators about the impact on soldiers' ability to perform their jobs.

But at the time, meaningful data—if it did exist—was fragmented and hard to find, and it had to be integrated manually from different databases. So, between 2012 and 2014, the Army system-level team built the digital infrastructure and analytics to gather data and display metrics on an electronic platform that was easily accessible to anyone in the Department of Defense. This gave department leaders like Lieutenant Colonel Johnson access to graphs and charts that had already been produced at the system level. Furthermore, because performance metrics were made freely available, it became possible for members of Johnson's department to log on to look at their performance data at any time. This set of centrally calculated and easily accessed metrics was an essential step in building the behavioral health performance management system.

Second, an effective performance management system depended on a clear and coherent leadership organization. Without clear lines of authority between levels of the system, knowledge could not be reliably transferred from one part of the organization to another. Insights gained from the performance management process would need to be turned into action at the local level, and system leaders would need to hold local leaders accountable.

As chapter 3 describes, the Army formed service lines that created lines of communication between behavioral health leaders at the clinic level and those at the system level. The service lines also enabled system-level leaders to engage and get assistance from other experts working in the headquarters, such as when facility modifications were needed or when information technology experts were needed to solve a problem impeding behavioral health care at the local level. The service lines also eliminated competing lines of authority, such as those created by discipline-specific departments of psychiatry, psychology, and social work. The service lines took shape and formed a major piece that was required to translate lessons learned at the system level into tangible changes in care delivery at the local level.

Third, successful performance management also needed engaged leaders at all levels, but especially local leaders in the hospitals and clinics. (In chapter 8 we detail the critical importance of leaders throughout a learning behavioral health system.) The performance management process places particular demands on leaders to ensure that a culture (whether of an entire organization or its components) embraces, or at least accepts, change. From the perspective of a clinic leader or individual provider, performance management involves not just measuring processes and outcomes, but also exposing that information to leaders at higher levels in the system and to peers in other hospitals and clinics. Leaders set the culture and, in doing so, determine, to a large degree, whether a performance management system will succeed.

The Army's investment in reliable, centrally managed data, a clear and coherent leadership organization at the highest level, and engaged leaders at the local level were the preconditions that set the stage for it to build a coherent performance management system.

Designing the Army Performance Management System

The Army refined its approach to performance management over several years of trial and error, keeping practices and metrics that worked and discarding those that didn't. Today, the Army health system uses data about the care it has recently delivered, including the quality of that care, to improve care that will be delivered in the future. In the Army's view, performance management encompasses the implementation of new administrative or clinical practices and incorporates many functions that are sometimes managed separately. Performance management brings the learning process to life. It's *how* an organization actually learns.

Today's Army performance management system includes three major parts, which facilitate the learning process used by leaders at all levels. The components are establishing a foundation of clinical outcome metrics, using metrics to inform changes to process, and implementing those changes to care delivery. These served as a helpful framework for the Army as it worked to gain oversight of the efficiency and effectiveness of its behavioral health clinics.

A Foundation of Clinical Outcome Metrics

In 2018, Lieutenant Colonel Smith—the chief of a department of behavioral health in a large Army hospital—sat down with the administrative and clinical leaders in her department, including psychiatrists, psychologists, and social workers, for their monthly performance review. She began the meeting by logging on to a website run by the behavioral health team at the system level. She clicked on her hospital's name and saw the four top-priority metrics that had been designated at the system level. The page displayed data that were specific to the health of the patients treated in her hospital and the performance of her clinical teams applied against the same standard used across all Army hospitals. In fact, if Smith wanted to compare her team's performance against similar facilities, she could have viewed the data from any Army hospital just by clicking on its name.

Lieutenant Colonel Smith decided to stay focused on her facility and selected the first of the top-tier metrics: "Treatment Response of Patients with Post-Traumatic Stress Disorder." The next screen displayed how many patients her providers had diagnosed with PTSD in the last six months and, of those, how many had improved by a significant degree. Lieutenant Colonel Smith and her administrative and clinical leaders noticed that their performance in this area was lagging behind the average of other Army hospitals, which was also displayed on the graph.

Army leaders, as the example above shows, manage behavioral health very differently than they did in 2010. First and foremost, they now have the ability to examine how effectively their teams perform their core mission: reducing the symptoms of mental illnesses in their patients, also known as clinical outcome data or measurement-based care. In 2010, clinical outcome data, which in behavioral health care is usually based on standardized questionnaires filled out by the patients that categorize and quantify symptoms of their mental health conditions, were not even routinely collected. Like most other health care system providers, the Army could only attempt to infer the effectiveness of its behavioral health care by measuring processes, such as how quickly patients received an outpatient appointment after being discharged from an inpatient ward or how soon appointments were available for new patients. It was like a coach trying to determine how good his football team was without being able to keep score of the games.

By implementing the Behavioral Health Data Portal (BHDP), the automated method for collecting, displaying, and aggregating clinical outcome data, the Army rapidly became a national leader in measurement-based care for outpatient mental health.[5] The Army could determine how frequently groups of patients reached established thresholds of clinical improvement—in other words, it could keep score of the games. It was an unparalleled opportunity to build a completely different type of performance management system, one based on the outcome of the care the Army provided.

The use of clinical outcome measures in the performance management process is not as uniformly accepted in behavioral health care as one might suppose. In fact, to use the exciting new data coming from the BHDP, the Army had to wrestle with a thorny issue known as the *case mix problem*, which impedes many health care systems from making use of clinical outcomes. The heart of the challenge is that the patients who receive care in one clinic are never exactly the same as patients receiving care in other clinics and hospitals—something true in any health care system that serves different populations in different locations. In all sorts of health care systems, some patients have more severe symptoms than others. Some are older, some may be more frequently homeless, some lack supportive families, and so on. Many of these differences have a direct effect on how frequently patients will recover from a behavioral health problem. A clinic that happens to have a higher proportion of "tougher" patients may look much less effective in its outcome metrics than a clinic with a higher proportion of "easier" patients, even though there may be no difference in the quality of the care they deliver.

To use clinical outcome metrics to figure out which clinics were delivering the best care, the Army had to account for the case mix problem. The Army began by gauging the actual size of the case mix issue. It compared the number and severity of each type of mental health condition by patients in each hospital. Fortunately, the distribution between clinics was much smaller than had been reported by other health care systems. Most Army clinics had about the same proportion and severity of patients with depression, PTSD, and other conditions, which made sense. The Army is a relatively homogenous group of people who meet specific eligibility requirements to join, and once in the Army, all have jobs, homes, and predictable paychecks—characteristics that may be part of the case mix problem in civilian health care systems. Many are exposed to similar stressors, such as moving frequently and deploying into combat.

While the Army's case mix problem didn't look as perplexing as in other health care systems, there were differences that still needed to be accounted for. To do that, the Army designed its clinical outcome metric so that achieving a "positive" response when treating a patient with a mild or severe mental health problem would be equally likely across all clinics. For example, if Corporal Ortega presented for treatment with depression, he could be counted as a "positive" response if his symptoms decreased by ten points as measured on the Patient Health Questionnaire (PHQ-9), a standard scale for symptoms of depression, or if he scored 7 or lower. After a course of treatment, patients with severe depression (and high initial PHQ-9 scores) were more likely to have a drop of ten points and patients with mild depression (and low initial PHQ-9 scores) were more likely to score a 7 or below. Providers treating patients at both ends of the spectrum of severity had a reasonable chance to help them improve enough to reach the metric's threshold. Such a design addressed most providers' concerns about the case mix problem.

Changing the Process to Improve the Outcome

Lieutenant Colonel Smith's department meeting continued. She wanted to understand why her department was not performing as well as other Army hospitals in getting its patients with PTSD better. She clicked on another tab on the same website to view more detailed metrics that related specifically to her department's patients with PTSD. Those metrics showed her that her providers were actually well ahead of other hospitals in two areas: how frequently they used BHDP and how their patients rated their level of engagement during treatment (also called "therapeutic alliance").

"Obviously," Smith told her team, we don't need to focus on these areas. But we're way below the Army average on how frequently our PTSD patients return to treatment for at least four visits, is well below the Army average—so let's work on that." Had that been the end of the meeting—Smith simply instructing her clinic chiefs to improve their performance on the PTSD clinical outcome metric by getting their patients better more quickly—she would have been met with exasperation. You can't improve an outcome simply by telling your subordinates to do so. An extension of our sports comparison may help to make the point. Our football coach would be foolish to expect his team to win a game just because he told them to score more points than the other team. Good coaches, like good leaders, change something about the process their team is using when they're after improvements. A football team, for instance, may practice longer, adopt a different pregame routine, or change up the plays it uses during the game itself.

But Lieutenant Colonel Smith did not end the meeting with that simple admonition to work on being better. Instead, she and her team spent the next hour clicking through more detailed data on the Army website that related to the problem of not getting soldiers with PTSD in for appointments frequently enough. Knowing that they were lagging behind other hospitals was only motivation for the clinic chiefs to improve, not information that could help them change anything. The clinic chiefs were *already* doing everything they knew to do to treat their patients' mental health conditions as effectively as possible. Clearly, they needed to know what to do *differently*.

To help focus leaders' time and energy on things they could directly control—process steps—the Army built a second group of metrics describing specific steps in the treatment process known to be associated with good clinical outcomes. These became the highest-priority metrics. Because this second group of metrics was intended to "drive" improved clinical outcomes, the system-level team came to call this group of metrics "drivers." They identified the drivers by analyzing the clinical outcome data produced through BHDP and looking for correlations between patients that improved and actions the clinical teams had taken as part of those improved patients' treatment.

Four drivers were found for depression and PTSD, the two most common and serious behavioral health conditions found in soldiers: (1) patients returned for treatment at least three times in the first ninety days after their initial visit; (2) providers documented that they used an evidence-based treatment; (3) patients rated highly their provider's therapeutic alliance with them during the treatment process; and (4) providers used BHDP when delivering care for the patient. Identifying these drivers for leaders at the local level—department chiefs such as Lieutenant Colonel Smith and her clinic chiefs—provided insight into specific, actionable steps teams could take that would have a direct impact on improving the care being provided to their patients.

Today, the Army's system-level team continually analyzes these data, looking for evidence of new drivers.

Understanding Process Problems

As the meeting continues, Lieutenant Colonel Smith wonders aloud, "How bad is our staffing problem? Maybe that's why we're having trouble bringing our patients in for follow-up visits?" She clicks over to the staffing metric, which shows that her department has about 15 percent fewer clinical staff than the minimum number recommended by the system-level team. She then opens the associated digital tool, colloquially called the "matrix," that breaks down the minimum staffing requirement for each clinic and helps her pinpoint where providers may be needed most in her department.

"Where are we on getting the new staff on board?" Smith asks Dane, her lead administrator, seeking an update on each hiring action currently in process. The entire team then discusses refocusing attention on the most critical vacancies on the list. The data made available by the system-level team will clearly support her request for additional staff and help with the approval she'll need from her budget-conscious hospital commander.

Smith and her team click through several other metrics related to the challenges they face in seeing patients with PTSD as frequently as they'd like. They're searching for other insights into the problems that make it more difficult to do what's necessary to help patients recover from their behavioral health conditions. The meeting ends with Smith and her team all agreeing on a short list of actions they'll take in the next month to treat soldiers with PTSD more effectively.

The metrics Lieutenant Colonel Smith and her team were reviewing were a third group the Army developed—practice management metrics—to help leaders at the local level gain insight into *why* their teams were having problems performing critical steps in the treatment process. Sometimes, the reasons are primarily administrative in nature, such as a shortage of clinical staff. Smith's team validated their concern that they could not offer sufficient appointments for soldiers with PTSD due to a lack of providers in their clinic with an objective staffing metric using a system-wide standard based on an analysis of the demand for behavioral health care of their specific beneficiary population. As a result, Lieutenant Colonel Smith's decision in 2018 to pursue additional hiring actions was informed by data, a stark contrast to Lieutenant Colonel Johnson's situation in 2010.

This third group of metrics also includes information about how frequently patients leaving inpatient care are seen in outpatient clinics within set time frames and how often hospitals are incorporating telehealth technology, as well as information about other administrative areas of the practice. Each metric is intended to provide local leaders with insights into their clinical operations from a different angle.

While these metrics are infrequently used by system-level leaders, because they are too detailed and affected by local factors to be used as system-wide performance measures, they are proving valuable at the local level as department and clinic chiefs seek to understand why their clinics are performing in certain ways.

Managing Performance at the System Level

At the system level, the behavioral health service line team played several important roles. Chief among them was to develop the overall metric plan, which included designing, prioritizing, and attaching incentives to achieving specific goals on some metrics. The team strived to make data useful for leaders at the local level so they could use it to inform decision making, and so the metrics supported learning by clinic and department chiefs. That meant the data had to be updated frequently, generally monthly, and be viewable at the department level and, when possible, even the clinic or provider level. The system-level team members, who had worked at the department level before the era of the service line, understood that local leaders could lead change only from a foundation of accurate, current, and detailed data with which to work.

The service line team at the system level also thought through the steps hospitals would have to take to implement major changes to its clinical programs that were necessary to reach the strategic goal of a learning behavioral health system with standardized clinical programs in each hospital. The system-level team then designed metrics to measure progress along the way (figure 6.2).

The most basic measures are structural metrics, which describe how effectively a hospital or clinic is putting the tangible pieces of a clinic or clinical program into place. These could include, among other things, the number of clinical staff hired by the hospital, the number of providers who have completed required training on a new therapeutic technique, or a count of new clinics constructed. These measures help leaders such as Lieutenant Colonel Smith to know whether she has enough providers hired and trained and sufficient space in her clinics from which to work. In our football analogy, structural metrics are akin to the coach counting the number of players he has on the field.

Process metrics describe how individual providers or clinical teams are operating. These measures include the number of patients seen, RVUs produced, types of treatment performed, and other quantifiable actions. Process metrics let Lieutenant Colonel Smith know how long patients have to wait until they can access the clinic, how frequently providers deliver therapeutic interventions to them, and how well providers are documenting the care they provide. They are like the coach,

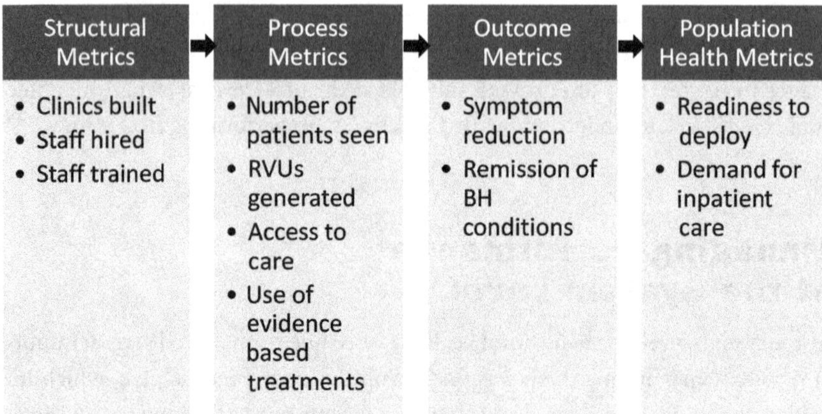

FIGURE 6.2. Aligning metrics with system development

once the team is on the field, assessing how well the players throw a forward pass, tackle the opponent's players, or kick field goals.

In behavioral health care, clinical outcome metrics are the most commonly aggregated patient-reported data. In the Army, clinical outcome metrics are collected through BHDP and used as part of the measurement-based care effort. Clinical outcome metrics indicate how patients' symptoms change through the course of treatment and provide a powerful mechanism for individual providers to modify their treatment approaches. When aggregated, clinical outcome metrics let leaders know which clinical teams, programs, or even entire hospitals are most effectively delivering care. They are the football coach looking at the scoreboard at the end of the game to see whether his team won the game.

They are also important indicators for the next game. They help leaders know whether there are structural or process problems that need to be addressed. Lieutenant Colonel Smith realized that her staffing problem (a structure metric) was likely contributing to her clinics' challenges in getting patients in for four visits in ninety days (a process metric), which was negatively affecting patients' recovery from PTSD (a clinical outcome metric).

Finally, population health metrics quantify the impact of behavioral health conditions, such as the inpatient bed days required to address behavioral health conditions and the prevalence of behavioral health conditions during unit-wide screening. These measures build on clinical outcome metrics, because as leaders such as Lieutenant Colonel Smith improve structures, processes, and outcomes of treating PTSD, for example, the impact of untreated PTSD in the population should decrease. Patients should require fewer days in the hospital, because they're more effectively treated as outpatients.

The system-level team also understood the importance of prioritizing specific metrics, which is necessary to help local leaders take actions that move their organizations toward goals established at the system level. Like Lieutenant Colonel Smith, department chiefs have multiple ways to solve a problem, but each option changes the organization, even if only in a small way. For instance, hiring an additional provider expands access to care but also increases overall payroll—meaning there is both a positive and negative impact. Similarly, increasing the number of patients a provider must see each day expands access to care, but it may risk burning out the clinical staff and heightens the chance staff may leave the organization to work elsewhere.

Lieutenant Colonel Smith and others in similar positions must determine how each course of action affects the organization's priorities, but to do so they need to know what those priorities are. With a good understanding of what the organization values most, the local leader can make decisions with confidence that leaders at the system level will support those decisions, because although there may be some trade-offs in terms of negative impacts, the decisions are seen as moving the organization in the right direction.

To communicate the Army's priorities to leaders at the local level, the system-level team created tiers of metrics based on level of importance. The four highest-priority metrics in tier 1 were determined to be the most critical in that particular year to advancing the organization toward its goals. To reinforce their importance, local and regional leaders were required to report regularly on their performance to the Army surgeon general and other executive leaders. The system-level team also created financial incentives for each tier 1 metric. The better a hospital performed, the greater the funding the hospital would receive.

In 2018, it was clear to everyone in the organization what the priorities were.

Lessons for Other Health Systems

Most of the academic and practice literature on mental health performance management focuses on decisions at the provider level because there are few integrated delivery systems that include mental health care. Even systems that have achieved some degree of integration, such as the Veterans Health Administration, have not developed methods to collect clinical outcome metrics systematically and use them in the performance management process across the enterprise. The recent manual from the Substance Abuse and Mental Health Services Administration (SAMHSA) on measures for behavioral health identifies thirty-two provider-level measures of care quality, but leaves it to individual organizations to figure out how those metrics can be aggregated to enable clinic, hospital, and health system decision making.[6] A majority of the CMS measures are structure and process measures that do not incorporate patient-reported outcomes, reflecting the current state of mental health care delivery in the United States.

The Army's performance management system supports decision making by executives, hospital and clinic leaders, and providers. The metrics used to assess performance are based on actual clinical care delivered, allowing for a tiered system of metrics to be established.

Measurement-based care is still in its infancy in mental health care practice management.[7] Many systems still rely on measures of structure and process as substitutes for assessing effectiveness. Some studies have concluded that clinicians who have their patients complete standardized questionnaires throughout treatment get better results than those that do not, while others have found much less benefit.[8] It takes time and persistence to routinize the collection of patient-reported outcome measures. Recent research has shown that more than 65 percent of the time, providers collect patient-reported outcomes at least once, but continued use of routine outcome measurements drops significantly, to less than 40 percent, when it comes to consistent collection over multiple visits.[9] Establishing the needed infrastructure and resources to support routine outcome data collection can take a long time; in Australia, just such an effort took more than ten years.[10]

To the Army's credit, its clinicians since 2015 have routinely collected patient-reported outcome data on more than 80 percent of all eligible outpatient visits. The Army experience shows not only that routine collection of patient-reported data is achievable, but also that the process can be accelerated by a learning behavioral health system.

The Army supplements the clinical outcome data with productivity and case mix data so clinicians can see the administrative aspects of care delivered. All Army providers can use the CART tool described in chapter 5 to assess their own productivity, determine whether they are meeting standards, and see how they compare to their peers in other locations. This also creates an empirical basis for talent management and year-end performance assessments that have to be carried out by clinic chiefs and other hospital leaders.

The metrics the Army uses to assess clinical productivity are easily replicable by other systems (in fact, most systems only measure some sort of *provider* productivity). What the Army has done is provide transparency regarding how those metrics are calculated.

Tools for sharing provider productivity information have value for any behavioral health care system. The consistent use of routine outcome measurement simplifies case mix analysis significantly, so clinic chiefs can make empirically informed arguments to help providers improve their performance.

A standardized digital infrastructure and transparent provider productivity assessment also allows the Army to assess its spending on care. Today, behavioral health leaders can instantly access their year-to-date spending and compare their performance to that of their peers in other hospitals.

The Army now manages the performance of its mental health system based on the actual clinical care delivered. It incorporates the analytics tools discussed in chapter 5 to allow providers, clinic leaders, hospitals, and the Army as a whole to make better decisions to improve the patient experience of care and care quality. As the Army has fully implemented the mental health system of care, the performance management system has also evolved. It began with a focus on the structure and process metrics to examine whether the foundations of sufficient providers and the right clinics existed to provide the needed care. Over time, the performance management system could be refined to focus on whether patient outcomes were improving, and whether the care itself was patient centered. The Army approach provides the template other health systems can replicate.

Chapter 7

CREATING DISSEMINATION AND IMPLEMENTATION CAPABILITIES

January 21, 2012, at the Pentagon was an overcast Saturday that had begun with light, freezing rain. General Peter Chiarelli, the vice chief of staff of the Army, gathered many of the Army's most senior leaders into a conference room. Dozens of others joined via videoconference from posts around the world. "The Vice," as he was called, wanted them to hear the MIT team's assessment of behavioral health care delivery in the Army.

At General Chiarelli's direction several months earlier, the MIT team had visited eight posts and talked with more than 220 people in the first round of visits to understand how the Army could improve the behavioral health care it provided. The team relayed its sobering conclusion that the high demand for behavioral health care had exceeded Army hospitals' capacity to provide care, and the Army was paying a steep price.

Soldiers faced significant delays getting into care, and when they finally reached it, that care was fragmented and poorly coordinated. Hospitals often resorted to triaging patients by using most of their available clinical resources to resolve mental health *crises* in soldiers experiencing them, which left precious little for other patients in need of more routine outpatient treatment. Unit leaders were also unhappy with the difficulties they faced when trying to discuss concerns with behavioral health providers, such as whether their soldier would be able to deploy or needed additional support. Readiness—a combat unit's ability to deploy to war—was suffering because commanders didn't know which soldiers could deploy and which soldiers needed to stay home due to serious behavioral health problems.

The Vice wasn't surprised by the report—he had heard similar stories from his subordinate leaders—but hearing it all together in a report from across the Army motivated him more than ever to find ways to fix the problems.

Despite the overall grim assessment, the MIT team did report some good news. Among the posts the team had visited, Fort Carson in Colorado stood out as an exception. Employing the Embedded Behavioral Health (EBH) model of outpatient care developed there, Fort Carson had succeeded in overcoming many of the problems that plagued other Army posts. Leaders there had moved ten- to thirteen-person teams of behavioral health staff out of the large hospital and into newly built or renovated clinics located within walking distance of where soldiers lived and worked. Within each EBH team, individual behavioral health providers matched up with individual Army combat units so that all soldiers assigned to that unit and in need of behavioral health care would start with the same provider. EBH providers also established working relationships with the leaders in combat units to develop ways units could support each soldier's recovery. That was what happened with Sergeant Chavez, a senior supply sergeant who was dealing with recurrent PTSD symptoms from his last deployment to Iraq.

Sergeant Chavez's behavioral health provider was very happy with the skills the soldier had developed for managing those PTSD symptoms over six months of treatment sessions in the EBH clinic. When one day Chavez said that his unit was getting ready for a field training exercise, the provider wasn't concerned. "I've put him on a duty-limiting profile with weapons restrictions," he thought to himself, "so he shouldn't have to go into the field." But then Chavez surprised him. "Doc," he said, "I don't want my guys to go without me. I know you're not going to be there in the field with us, and I'm going to be in the suck [soldier slang for undesirable conditions], but I should be there to make my guys successful."

In a different setting, the provider's response would have been predictable pushback. The provider would have acknowledged Sergeant Chavez's desire to be with his "guys" while making clear the reason he was "on a profile"—that he was not currently deployable. But that was the old setting, where the provider didn't know anything about Chavez's role as a supply sergeant or didn't have an understanding of the unit culture. However, in the first six months of EBH implementation, the provider had already met three times with Chavez's battalion commander. The first time was when the provider joined the EBH team and went to the battalion commander's office to introduce himself as the EBH team member who would be taking care of his soldiers. The second time was when the battalion commander, Lieutentant Colonel Greg, saw that Sergeant Chavez was placed on a duty-limiting profile that included weapons restrictions. The battalion commander wanted to make sure to share his thoughts with the provider, so he stopped by the EBH clinic to let the provider know that Chavez was a great soldier who had been under fire in Iraq, and that he (the battalion commander) would do whatever was necessary to make sure that Chavez was able to recover. The third time was at the battalion commander's "high-risk meeting," a monthly meeting the commander held at which he, along with his subordinate commanders and key experts such as the EBH provider, reviewed all the soldiers who were on a duty-limiting profile, including Chavez.

So, having established this relationship with the battalion commander in settings different than what had been typical in the past, the provider felt comfortable telling Chavez he would talk to the battalion commander about the possibility of making changes to his profile.

We asked the provider to tell us about the call he had with Lieutenant Colonel Greg, the battalion commander.

> I called and told him Sergeant Chavez wanted to go on the field exercise. His first question was, "Doc, is it good for him to be in the field? When you put him on profile with weapons restrictions, you told us you were working on his startle response. You also wanted to make sure he was getting enough sleep at night. The field exercises will definitely disrupt his sleep!"
>
> I explained to the commander that Sergeant Chavez was no longer on sleep meds, and that he could go to the field, but that I was still worried about immersing him fully in the battle environment.
>
> Lieutenant Colonel Greg immediately said, "Doc, I can put him in the TOC [tactical operations center]. That way, he's not fully exposed but will still be able to do his job and support the team. But how do I take a guy to the field with a weapons restriction? We're going to be in full battle rattle—he has to have his weapon with him."
>
> I asked him whether he could just pull the firing pin from the weapon if he was going to have Chavez in the TOC. No one else needs to know that, I said, and I would be more comfortable in letting him join the field training exercise. Lieutenant Colonel Greg agreed, and Sergeant Chavez was able to join his unit in the field exercise.

Collaboration of that sort between a behavioral health provider and the commander to shape soldier recovery was exceedingly rare before the implementation of EBH. Fort Carson had bridged a divide that existed on almost every other large Army post at the time. Soldiers there got care more quickly; commanders received better communication about the ability of their soldiers to deploy; and readiness improved.[1]

The MIT team's presentation convinced General Chiarelli that EBH would help address many of the behavioral health problems facing the Army, and he ordered the Army Medical Command to implement it in all its hospitals.[2] Suddenly, Army medical leaders found themselves faced with a monumental task: transform how their hospitals delivered outpatient behavioral health care to soldiers by implementing an entirely new clinical program that required new physical structures, an expanded workforce, new training programs, and revised administrative and business processes. The members of the small behavioral health leadership team working at the Army level knew they had their work cut out for them.

A mandate to implement sweeping change isn't something unique to the Army. Health care systems in the civilian world continually seek to improve the care they offer by identifying and disseminating new clinical practices—often creating daunting challenges with their mandates. For instance, Dr. Delos "Toby" Cosgrove, then president and CEO of Cleveland Clinic, spoke in 2010 about required changes to the hospital's integrated delivery system resulting from a shift in the center of gravity away from hospitals to outpatient and home care settings.[3] But five years later, Cleveland Clinic leaders were still grappling with the challenge of transforming a health care system known for being great at treating the "sickest of the sick" to building capabilities in primary care and chronic condition management.[4]

The Department of Veterans Affairs (VA) has had significant success in implementing its primary care–centered strategy to improve access and quality of veteran mental health care. The VA had been compelled to take its steps by, in part, research showing that integrating behavioral health care in the primary care setting increased communication between providers, reduced stigma for patients, and made for better care coordination for its patient population.[5] In 2004, the VA developed a five-year mental health strategic plan that centered on implementing mental health care in primary care settings.[6]

The Veterans Administration had identified three different approaches within VA health centers for integrating mental health in primary care. One was the Behavioral Health Laboratory that was developed at the Philadelphia VA, in which primary care providers could request that a telephonic assessment be made by a behavioral health care provider.[7] The Translating Initiative in Depression into Effective Solutions (TIDES) approach was another; in TIDES, a patient was referred to a co-located depression care nurse manager, who would coordinate the patient's care with the mental health care provider and manage the collaboration between the primary care provider and the behavioral health care provider(s).[8] A third model, developed at the White River Junction VA in Vermont, focused on co-locating behavioral health care providers as members of the primary care team itself.[9] These models differed in their requirements for staff, changes to clinician workflows, and changes to patient flows within the primary care clinic.

The VA initially allowed primary care practices within VA facilities to select the model best suited for that facility. Unsurprisingly, there was large variation across different primary care practices, with one assessment of 225 VA primary care practices finding that almost half the sites (107) had chosen to implement the White River Junction model, while only seventeen had implemented the BHL.[10] The VA developed a standardized model that incorporated key features such as co-located collaborative care (from the White River Junction model) and care management (from TIDES and BHL), and also published a manual to help guide implementation efforts.[11]

Today, all primary care clinics in the Veterans Administration have some form integrated behavioral health care. The VA found that successful implementations shared four things in common: they had strong implementation infrastructure, implementation leadership, standardized clinical workflows, and adequate staff.[12] The Army incorporated the lessons learned from the VA's efforts to improve the implementation of Embedded Behavioral Health in the Army.

Small-scale changes such as using a new metric or retraining existing clinical staff can pose some implementation challenges, but those can typically be handled by existing leadership teams. Large-scale changes with multiple component parts, such as transforming how outpatient clinics are organized, are another story; leadership teams often struggle because they have to juggle many specific change efforts (all linked to the larger objective) simultaneously. Learning health care systems overcome the problem by creating the dissemination and implementation capabilities to support leaders in making sweeping changes. They create a trusted source of knowledge about the change to be implemented, develop dissemination and implementation structures to teach different stakeholders about the change, empower people, and allocate the resources needed to implement the change.

Early Struggles

Generals in command of Army posts around the world were in attendance at that meeting that ended with General Chiarelli's order to the Army surgeon general. They, too, heard the MIT team's description of the improvements EBH had made at Fort Carson, and many wanted it on their posts immediately. In the months that it would take the Army medical leadership to develop the capacity to manage EBH implementation, many posts launched efforts to build their own EBH clinics. Each encountered major problems that halted or slowed implantation. Their collective experience demonstrated why health care systems must have the ability to create and manage large-scale change.

The first posts that attempted to replicate EBH didn't have a clear picture of what EBH was or how it worked, and they lacked the resources to implement it.

On one post, the limiting factor was the lack of understanding. There, the chief of behavioral health had moved clinical staff into buildings closer to the combat units, but did not arrange them to support *specific* units, a key step in developing the kinds of working relationships that are so critical to EBH's success. On another post, EBH implementation was stymied by a lack of funding for facilities. The behavioral health chief there could not find a way to fund the small buildings he wanted to build to house EBH providers close to where soldiers work and live, and he ended up abandoning the effort altogether. All in all, the first attempts to replicate EBH were unsuccessful because system-level leaders did not yet have a way to provide the support of the system in terms of information, resources, and expertise to local leaders.

Informed by the early, ad hoc attempts to replicate EBH, the Army began to build capacity in the form of a small team to perform several core functions necessary to drive the change. That team provided the *definitive source of knowledge* about EBH, *active oversight of EBH implementation*, and *provider and leader training* in EBH. Over time, the team transitioned skills to individual hospitals *to make the change stick.*

A Definitive Source of EBH Knowledge

Army medical leaders established a three-person EBH program management office (PMO) within the behavioral health service line leadership team. All three brought deep Fort Carson experience to their new jobs. One of the authors of this book relocated from his position as Fort Carson's chief of the Department of Behavioral Health to the Army's Office of the Surgeon General in Falls Church, Virginia, to provide the overall leadership. The former lead administrator in that same department was reassigned to the PMO as the administrative lead; he had successfully navigated the administrative, financial, facility, and personnel-related challenges necessary to implement EBH at Fort Carson and would now support other hospitals to do the same. The third member of the PMO team was a psychologist who had led the first EBH team established at Fort Carson three years earlier; she took on the clinically related aspects of the initiative, based on her experience in establishing the clinical processes and treatment approaches in EBH clinics.

The PMO team went to work creating a definitive source of knowledge on EBH by writing two foundational documents. The first, the EBH concept of operations, was intended to inform leaders across the Army about EBH and generate their support for it; it explained the history, rationale, and benefits of the EBH model. The concept of operations also let the Army know that a clinical leadership team had been established to define and replicate a standard version of EBH and to reduce the chance that leaders would attempt to implement a different version.

The second document, the EBH operations manual, was designed to give local leaders specific information and tools needed to implement and manage EBH clinics. Every EBH clinic implemented according to the operations manual would have the same type and mix of providers: one prescriber per EBH team, one psychotherapist per battalion, and support staff, which would include at least one case manager, two behavioral health technicians, and two medical support assistants. These clinics would have shared workflows and offer the same evidence-based treatments.

Before the implementation of EBH, providers within each clinic chose their own treatment modalities, and there was no standard treatment pathway for a given condition. Depending on the provider a depressed soldier first saw in the clinic, she might have been treated with medications alone, individual psychotherapy, group psychotherapy, or some combination of medications and therapy. Only a few clinics were using group psychotherapy, even though demand for care was rising at a rate that made it impossible to meet the need without groups. Psychotherapists preferred one-on-one therapy sessions with soldiers, which they *felt* were better than group sessions. That provider preference had another driver: providers found it easier to meet their productivity targets using individual sessions because groups didn't generate as many RVUs per session, despite taking up the same amount of time. Plus, group sessions required more administrative work to close out notes for each participant. And from a practice management perspective, individual sessions made it easier for a clinic chief to compare productivity across providers. The result was significant variation from one clinic to the next in terms of both the treatments offered and the overall care of patients.

The EBH operations manual directly addressed that variation to make sure individual sessions were warranted. When a soldier first came in, either for a scheduled appointment or as a walk-in, the provider made a clinical decision regarding whether to assign that soldier to a group session. Groups are particularly appropriate for soldiers who have never before used behavioral health care, and so might be placed in an "introduction to behavioral health" group, or who need to develop coping skills for dealing with life stressors, such as in an anger management group. That simple change in patient flow meant care capacity was being used in a more optimal manner.

The manual also standardized communication pathways. The daily huddles now bring together the entire care team to build shared clinical situational awareness. Multidisciplinary treatment planning meetings help providers coordinate their care. All providers communicate with command teams electronically when a soldier has a duty-limiting behavioral health condition, using a system called E-Profile.

While standardization was the primary goal, the highly detailed manual did recognize that local leaders needed flexibility in some key areas, such as how to organize the team to support unconventional and unique Army units. For example, the 385th Military Police (MP) Battalion at Fort Stewart in Georgia is part of a larger MP brigade with battalions on four other installations. Using the manual, behavioral health leaders at Fort Stewart tailored the usual EBH team staffing model by creating a new EBH clinic to support all six separate battalions on the post. This clinic had only five providers, but the 385th MP Battalion was large enough that a provider was aligned to that battalion exclusively.

The EBH operations manual specified key workflows that affect mental health care delivery. In some cases, those workflows represented dramatic changes to how patients moved within the larger system of care. For example, as a response in early 2011 to skyrocketing requests for behavioral health appointments from multiple brigades returning from Iraq and Afghanistan, the hospital leadership decided to create a central triage clinic. Any soldier coming back from deployment could walk into that clinic and be seen by a provider that day, even if it meant sitting in the waiting room for hours. The problem with the centralized triage system was that providers responsible for the "usual source of care" either did not know their soldiers had received treatment or they received delayed notification of that treatment. Nor was the central triage clinic convenient for soldiers. EBH clinics overcame all three issues by creating walk-in care capability within an EBH clinic *itself.* The EBH manual clearly established the scope of walk-in care to be rapid assessment of safety and any referral for any additional services. In the specified workflow, a soldier walking into the clinic would complete a triage assessment and then see a behavioral health technician who would perform an initial assessment and staff the case with the walk-in provider, who in turn would decide the appropriate next steps. The hospital was able to shut down the triage clinic and move those assets into EBH clinics.

The manual provides key management artifacts such as provider templates and standard operating procedures for managing new workflows. EBH required that provider templates support new ways of working, including setting aside time for the key meetings that are needed for patient-level and clinic-level learning, such as the morning huddle, command engagement meetings, and multidisciplinary treatment planning meetings.

Figure 7.1 is an example of a template for an EBH psychotherapist, showing the regularly scheduled meetings (daily and weekly), training hours, and opportunities to engage command teams (in three hour-long meetings and two half-hour telephone consultations). The template shows the provider doing intakes for

Time	Monday	Tuesday	Wednesday	Thursday	Friday
730	Morning Huddle	Morning Huddle	Morning Huddle	Morning Huddle	Morning Huddle
0800	Command Meeting	SPEC/60	GROUP	TRAINING	Command Meeting
0830					
0900	SPEC/60	EST/60			Designated Walk-in Provider
0930					
1000	EST/60	GROUP	EST/60		
1030					
1100	EST/60		EST/60	SPEC/60	
1130					
	LUNCH	LUNCH	LUNCH	LUNCH	LUNCH
1300	EST/60	EST/60	Multi-Disciplinary Treatment Planning Meeting	EST/60	Designated Walk-in Provider
1330					
1400	EST/60	EST/60		EST/60	
1430			SPEC/60		
1500	EST/60	EST/60		Command Meeting	
1530			Command Teleconference		Command Teleconference
1600	ADMIN	ADMIN	ADMIN	ADMIN	ADMIN

FIGURE 7.1. Sample EBH psychotherapist template

four new patients each week (SPEC/60), thirteen follow-up appointments (EST/60), and two group therapy sessions. This particular provider also serves as the designated walk-in provider on Fridays.

EBH clinic chiefs can modify the template to meet their local needs, establishing their own meeting times and changing the workload mix (groups, intakes, follow-ups) based on a provider's skill and interests. The EBH team lead can create a provider schedule for all providers on the team, to designate a different walk-in provider each day. The template also establishes the operational rhythm of the clinic; in the figure 7.1 example, multidisciplinary treatment planning meetings are always scheduled for Wednesday afternoons. These management artifacts are critical for disseminating information about the right way to implement EBH.

Active Oversight of EBH Implementation

The Army surgeon general also functioned as the commanding general of the Army's Medical Command, the equivalent of the hospital system's CEO. Because the behavioral health leadership team, including the EBH PMO, served on the surgeon general's staff, they were expected to send directives—called "orders" in the Army—on her behalf. Having defined EBH in two key documents, the PMO developed the directive to instruct Army hospitals to implement it.

These orders required commanders of Army hospitals to execute the directive, unless they could provide a compelling reason not to do so. The PMO wrote and published the order for Army hospitals on all posts with combat units to implement EBH over a period of five years. The order included guidance on important areas, including milestones that each hospital had to meet.[13]

Over the five-year implementation of EBH, the PMO refined its policy guidance based on lessons it learned in each previous implementation phase. The executive order, the operational order, and its variants became the core authority documents that guided the Army's implementation of EBH. This made it possible for a behavioral health chief to shape Army senior leader expectations about when they should expect to see EBH clinics on their post. As one behavioral health chief pointed out, "When the division commander says I want EBH for everyone, I can now show him formal Army guidance on the required implementation schedule. He may still say I have to do it faster, but now I have authority documents I can use to have an honest conversation about the resources needed to meet his directives."

The EBH PMO developed and tracked measures of the implementation process itself. Before the implementation began, each hospital reported on its current state, identifying all the units on the installation and specifying which units would have an EBH clinic. This current-state assessment included the number of behavioral health providers on the post and helped create the baseline for tracking implementation progress.

Once implementation began, close monitoring by the PMO ensured that the process was successful. The PMO developed monthly reports that had to be submitted by the hospitals; these reports communicated the key elements of implementation, such as the number of providers in each clinic and whether the clinic was located within walking distance of soldiers' workplaces. The reports were closely scrutinized by the PMO and reviewed in monthly calls with each hospital—a high level of attention that helped bring problems to light early in the implementation process so the PMO could address them. For example, by the end of 2012, Army hospitals reported having implemented eighteen EBH clinics, but those clinics only had eighty-five of the 126 providers needed to be fully staffed. Leaders in the PMO revised the reporting requirement to capture whether an EBH clinic was actually *functional*, defined as having at least three clinicians, a case manager, the needed support staff, and accurate documentation of administrative data. The new reporting requirement increased hospital leaders' attention to accurate, requisite staffing, resulting in twenty-eight new hires in the following year—which in turn made another five EBH clinics fully functional.

To augment its routine oversight from afar, the EBH PMO established a two-day site assistance visit program. PMO team members would visit Army hospitals to assess and support implementation efforts. The first day included a walk-through of each EBH clinic and focus groups with hospital and behavioral health leadership, unit leaders, and the EBH team members, often without the clinic chief or behavioral health leadership in the room. These activities gave the team an opportunity to see implementation through the eyes of the people most directly involved. On the second day, the team worked with the behavioral health leadership on the post to develop a plan to address any problems that had been uncovered.

The site visits proved to be an extremely useful way to understand the roots of problems facing local leaders. At one Army post, the reports submitted to the PMO showed that EBH implementation was significantly behind schedule. The post had enough clinicians to staff the required number of clinics, but those clinics weren't being opened. As the PMO team drove through the post, it became clear that the post actually had five clinics located within walking distance of the soldiers' workplaces—one for each of the brigade combat teams and one "all others" clinic for supporting other operational units—but they just weren't EBH clinics. They weren't organized in the manner required by the EBH manual, did not use standard clinical practices, and didn't bother to complete the monthly EBH report.

The team stopped at the behavioral health clinic, which was located on the second floor of a small building that was not being used by the brigade the EBH clinic supported. In the conversation, the story of the building emerged. It was located on a small hillock, with no road or even a footpath to get to it. Once upon a time, the brigade used it temporarily to store odds and ends, but those were eventually moved into shipping containers closer to the unit's headquarters building. Now, providers complained that soldiers had no idea where the clinic was, and even those who knew its location missed their appointments because they had no place to park their vehicles at the bottom of the hill. Providers had to use a small parking lot at the base of the hillock and walk up through the mud and roots to get to the building.

The physical problems with the building and its location told only part of the story. The clinic itself was not staffed fully: the psychiatrist was shared with another team, for example, and was only on site at the clinic two days a week. Asked why, the psychiatrist explained to the PMO team that the behavioral health chief had said the clinic didn't have enough demand to support a full-time prescribing provider. It was clear that no one was happy with the situation: providers weren't happy; the command team wasn't happy; the behavioral health leaders weren't happy. It was another example of why the PMO site visits were so important, giving the team insights into the lived experience of the actors involved in EBH implementation. In this case, the team members spoke with everyone and gained a deeper understanding of how patients flowed through the system.

When the team sat down with the behavioral health leadership team the following morning, it became clear that the behavioral health chief did not believe EBH was the right model for his post and had resisted implementation. "We have one of the lowest utilization rates for mental health as it is," he pointed out, "and my providers are being told to constantly do more work. Now you're asking me to move my providers to these remote clinics, where I can't see them or manage their productivity?!" The PMO team spent the next several hours reviewing the evidence supporting the EBH model. They showed him the actual data from the post on provider productivity, using the CART tool, and explained how he could use those data to assist his providers in meeting their productivity targets. The face-to-face interactions also allowed the team to work with the chief to allay his multiple concerns and convinced him to take a series of actions to implemented EBH on the post.

By the end of 2014, the Army had implemented thirty-six EBT teams staffed with 258 clinicians. The implementation framework had matured and the PMO had developed a deep understanding of the common modes of implementation failure, such as lack of facilities, insufficient number of providers, poor electronic health record connectivity, and lack of understanding of the EBH model.

As the implementation progressed, the monthly telephone conferences between the PMO and the local EBH leaders remained critical for identifying and resolving problems that were getting in the way of implementation. The PMO described the timing and details of telephone conferences as follows: "We would do the conference calls as soon as the Situational Reports came in. If no one on the call was asking questions, we would ask them questions about their reports. Usually we probed deeper when we saw inconsistencies between the reports and the PMO's own analysis of an installation's implementation. This helped the installations see themselves through both their own data and our analysis."

During one call, EBH clinic chiefs expressed their concerns about provider attrition during the first six months of running an EBH clinic. The empirical data analyzed by the PMO showed support for their concerns, so when the final revision of the operational order was published at the end of 2015, the PMO revised the situational report to capture explicitly the number of providers who had completed the EBH provider training course.

By 2016, the Army had fully implemented EBH to all operational units, and as of 2017 there were sixty-two fully functional Army EBH clinics staffed with 460 clinicians. The EBH PMO provided active and engaged oversight for EBH implementation to reach the goal of sixty-two clinics. The team's work would continue as the PMO learned more about the problems EBH clinics encountered.

Training Leaders and Providers on EBH

Many of the challenges in EBH implementation fell into two categories: clinic chiefs did not know how to manage EBH clinics, and providers did not understand the new EBH workflows.

So, leaders had to be trained on managing their clinics—which is a challenge because these leaders are providers first, and often do not have an appetite for management. The Army's approach to clinic management is tool driven, but these leaders did not grow up in the Army health system using such computer-based tools.

It was up to the PMO to make the training for leaders appealing and enduring. To accomplish that, the EBH PMO created two courses. One focused on training EBH leaders on the tools they needed to use in day-to-day management of their EBH clinics—and the Army made an important decision that no clinicians could take on the EBH chief role unless they completed that course. The other was a provider course to train clinicians on working in EBH clinics. It was created to address known challenges in providing culturally competent care, which requires understanding the social and occupational context for a soldier's behavioral health condition—like the provider in the Sergeant Chavez example provided earlier.

One EBH clinic chief told us just how valuable the provider training is—for uniformed providers (those who are service members) and civilian providers alike—to the success of EBH:

> I have uniformed providers that don't really know how the Army functions. They are all skilled clinicians, but they don't come equipped out of their clinical [graduate medical education] programs knowing how to assess readiness from a mission perspective, how to talk to command teams, or even how to deal with the military exception to [the federal health privacy law] HIPAA. If that's the case of a uniformed Army provider, just think about our civilians who come in with no understanding of *military* medicine. The provider training course fills that gap for me, so I don't have to train them. Once they complete the course, I can supervise and course correct. More importantly, I am not hearing con-

> stant complaints from command teams that my providers don't understand the Army.

A common complaint from early EBH implementation efforts concerned the challenge of dealing with walk-in patients. As one provider pointed out,

> I have three groups of soldiers that walk in. The first group is those in genuine distress, and I as a provider know exactly what to do. The second group is my singletons: they've had a bad day either at home or with the unit and just need someone to talk to for a little bit. The third group is soldiers who were told by their command or buddy to see someone at EBH. They don't really have an immediate concern and most have never seen behavioral health before. That third group is the hardest to deal with. What am I supposed to do with them? But now that we have EBH fully implemented, the soldiers in that third group go to the "introduction to behavioral health" group. Now walk-ins actually work!

Establishing an enduring training program overcame the two most common problems mentioned earlier that EBH teams faced: clinic chiefs not knowing how to manage EBH clinics, and providers not understanding the new EBH workflows. The PMO was the catalyst for creating the training program, locating the resources to establish it, and fine-tuning it over time.

Transferring Skills to Make Change Stick

After working through the many implementation challenges, the PMO focused on helping local leaders monitor and improve EBH without the direct intervention of system-level leaders. The Army's EBH implementation framework helped overcome the challenges faced by unprepared leaders, providers, and support staff. "We had a lot of clinically competent but managerially illiterate people, said one EBH chief, discussing what was learned from implementing EBH, "some of whom have embraced their illiteracy. The implementation framework adopted for rolling out EBH makes it very hard to remain incompetent or incapable. They are forced to build the managerial skills needed to understand and lead their local behavioral health system of care."

The EBH PMO designed reflexive learning processes to transfer skills to the individual hospitals to sustain EBH once full implementation was reached at the end of 2016. All operational orders have an "expiration date," the date by which leader guidance contained within an order is no longer enforced. The Army's expectation was that all hospitals would have fully implemented EBH, and that EBH was *the* way for delivering mental health care within walking distance of a soldier's workplace. Once there was no operational implementation order, the onus would be on the hospital to monitor internally whether EBH clinics were working.

At a 2018 off-site, the behavioral health leadership focused on how they could develop enduring authority documents. They found that the analytics tools the Army had developed for defining capacity, assessing productivity, and evaluating care effectiveness could also be used to analyze EBH implementation effectively. EBH clinic chiefs began to use the tools to gather data for the monthly situational reports on the progress of EBH implementation. The EBH PMO used the site assistance visits and the monthly conference calls to reinforce the skills taught in the EBH leader and provider training courses.

"If you had asked me four years ago with the legacy system if we could sustain something like EBH," one EBH clinic chief reflected, "the answer would have been no! But now, we can pull up the data on our own performance using the tools, compare performance against other clinics, and have the service line generate the metrics."

Lessons for Other Health Systems

Health systems struggle with systematic dissemination and implementation of innovation because they do not build the needed capabilities.

Dissemination capabilities focus on the targeted distribution of information and intervention materials to a specific audience.[14] This requires a single source of knowledge about the intervention and the target audience for the change.

The Army developed *a single source of knowledge* about each innovation being implemented. The EBH program management office published the authoritative documentation on EBH. The concept of operations document explains the rationale and expected impact of the innovation to key stakeholders who influence the implementation of the innovation and/or benefit from the innovation. The Army used the concept of operations to shape leaders' expectations about the impact of EBH on readiness, a key organizational outcome. This helped win leader support for key actions such as fencing off EBH funding to ensure successful and sustained implementation.

The EBH operations manual defines the roles and responsibilities of leaders, clinicians, and nonclinical actors, and specifies the common workflows associated with each role. Specifying the key roles within an EBH clinic greatly reduces misunderstandings about what the innovation is, how it should work, and who should be involved in the implementation and management of the innovation.

The Army *defined and updated policies supporting the implementation effort.* Well-written policy documents are the foundation of any implementation effort. The EBH PMO published six policy documents over the implementation life cycle, beginning with the publication of the operational order after General Chiarelli's executive order mandated the full implementation of EBH. The PMO revised the policy guidance based on lessons learned from site assistance visits, as well as from self-reported outcomes, to provide clear, consistent, and timely policy guidance.

"Implementation" is a broad term used to describe strategies used for the adoption and integration of evidence-based health interventions and associated changes to practice patterns within specific settings.[15] The Army's focus on specific clinical microsystems, such as EBH, meant that the implementation setting was clearly understood. The Army *invested implementation authority in one group within the organization*—the EBH program management office—and gave that office the authority to specify how EBH ought to be implemented on an Army post.

The EBH PMO identified key implementation levers such as staffing levels, staffing mix, facility size, and location, and standardized the collection of data on implementation levers through individual hospital reports. Reports on those key implementation levers are important for EBH chiefs, as one told us. "Our own tools help us in validating the numbers and triangulating data to see if the rollout is occurring to plan," he explained. "That also helps us see if we have functioning EBH teams. A recent report showed that our implementation was not to standard because we did not have enough EBH providers. But I know we have enough providers, so we dug deeper and saw that we had made a mistake in how we were assigning providers to administrative cost centers other than the actual EBH clinics. The report jump-started our analysis. Not only did we correct our own data, and get the report right, we actually were ahead of schedule in the implementation."

Implementation succeeds only if the people involved in doing the work know the changes that need to be made. The Army *trained providers and support staff in the new ways of working.* The Army actively identified and trained change agents within and across the Army. All EBH clinic chiefs were trained in a weeklong EBH leaders' course, where they worked with all the key management tools they would need to manage an EBH clinic. People were selected for these roles based on their leadership potential, and the clinic chief role is now seen as an important milestone in the overall career development of a provider.

The provider course included intensive training in small group settings on their roles and responsibilities within an EBH clinic, so that they could more easily adapt to the required new ways of working. "Providers come to this course with varying degrees of awareness and capacity," one of the instructors told us, highlighting the importance of small group work. "In some cases, it hasn't dawned on them that the entire model of care has changed and they need to change, too. In large groups, people don't want to ask any questions in front of their peers, but in small groups all the posturing falls away, and they leave with a much better understanding of EBH."

Tracking the degree to which the innovation is delivered as intended—the *implementation fidelity*—is critical.[16] The Army initially created specific reporting tools to track whether each clinical microsystem was being implemented as specified. While having specific reporting tools for individual clinical microsystems can be useful to start a change, the reporting requirements can quickly become an administrative burden. Over time, the Army transitioned to *using standard management tools to track implementation fidelity*. As the service line management tools such as the Distribution Matrix Tool and the Capacity Analysis and Reporting Tool (both described in chapter 5) were developed and standardized, they could be used to assess implementation fidelity. CART 2.0, for instance, was seen as a "godsend," as one leader explained: "I would have had to jump through hoops to get provider data from individual sites. Now I can break down all 517 providers, including behavioral health officers, and see which EBH clinics they work in."

Innovations often peter out when the high-level mandate for change disappears. In the EBH case, once the operations order expired, there was no requirement to implement EBH. The expectation was that EBH had become the new normal, and individual Army posts knew how to sustain it. The Army *created reflexive learning processes* to cement the capability of individual hospitals to oversee and improve EBH. The structured reporting and data collection enshrined within the EBH implementation policy are designed to help EBH clinic chiefs and providers learn about EBH and evaluate their own compliance to the standard of care it specifies. That said, routine reporting and monthly reflection do not always translate into learning. "I can measure a hospital's sustainment of progress based on where they are, against the implementation requirement for an EBH clinic," a leader observed. "I provided an EBH update a couple of weeks back where I had red and ambers all over the status—but only one person challenged my assessment! That was because that clinic chief could replicate my analysis using the standard enterprise tools."

Making bold changes to health care requires leaders to disrupt numerous components of the delivery system. Without reorganizing leaders to manage the process, those changes can be impossible to implement successfully. Learning behavioral health care systems empowers experts in the areas that require large-scale change to use their experience and expertise to lead the entire system through the change process. In doing so, they diffuse the innovation (no matter how large) through each of their clinics and hospitals so all patients benefit, no matter where they receive their care.

Chapter 8

LEADING A LEARNING SYSTEM

In 2014, about midway through the transformation, Chris's team in the Army medical headquarters (the system level) noticed a pattern of problems emerging at several Army hospitals that were struggling to make improvements at the same pace as the others. One of these hospitals—which provided care to soldiers and their families—came to the particular attention of the team because it failed to meet the benchmarks for implementing new clinical programs such as Embedded Behavioral Health clinics and intensive outpatient programs to treat soldiers with PTSD.

The hospital had determined it did not have the capacity to meet the clinical needs of many of its beneficiaries with mental health symptoms and was referring patients to other hospitals at a rate much higher than at similar-size facilities. The chief of the department of behavioral health was frustrated: her staff resisted potentially helpful changes of almost any kind, from moving offices to forming treatment teams with providers from disciplines other than their own (e.g., psychiatry, psychology, social work) or even participating in meetings to ensure close monitoring of high-risk patients. Several staff had filed formal complaints against the hospital leaders, citing a lack of proper reimbursement for the work they were asked to perform.

Chris's system-level team decided it had better pay the facility a visit and meet with local leaders and the clinical staff. It got an earful—and the reasons for the palpable frustration among providers and support staff became immediately clear.

First there was the issue of the facility itself. The clinic staff had been relocated twice in the previous several months, and many of the front desk staff had resigned to take jobs elsewhere. The moves and the support staff turnover had injected unpredictability into what should have been routine clinical operations. In the midst of the turmoil, three patients had committed suicide, landing a huge blow to providers' morale. Combat leaders, such as the commanders of the brigades on the post, were frustrated and losing faith in the effectiveness of behavioral health care; they believed the behavioral health team should have done more to prevent their soldiers' deaths.

When the system-level team dug deeper, they found out that the hospital had not standardized its position descriptions—the key personnel documents that specify the clinical duties and pay scales—to match the rest of the Army's hospitals, which meant some clinicians were being paid significantly less than they would earn elsewhere in the Army system. The perceived lack of equitable salaries eroded motivation to work and led providers to resist direction from their department chief to set up more clinics and offer intensive treatment options as required by system-level leaders. They viewed the data about implementing mandatory clinical programs and overuse of inpatient services as flawed or not applicable to their hospital's unique situation.

Providers also felt that the hospital had exposed them to undeserved blame from the combat unit leaders after the suicides, and for fear of attracting additional criticism, were resisting any changes to their traditional clinical practice. They acknowledged to the visitors that their patients were spending more time in inpatient and residential treatment programs than soldiers on similar posts, because they had begun to use a very low clinical threshold for admitting their patients to such programs to avoid the risk of more suicides. Being in these programs had stigmatizing and often career-threatening consequences for active-duty soldiers—recall the story in chapter 1 of the soldier carrying the large pink rock. Less stigmatizing programs such as Embedded Behavioral Health, which placed small outpatient clinics near soldiers' unit areas, or intensive outpatient programs that delivered several hours of treatment daily for several weeks without requiring a soldier to be admitted to the hospital, couldn't be implemented in the midst of the upheaval within the Department of Behavioral Health. The sides had dug in. Care remained stovepiped, disengaged from the soldiers and leaders it was intended to serve. Staff were resistant to making changes. Progress was not being made. The culture was toxic.

Fortunately, by this time in 2014, the Army had developed a method to measure each hospital's behavioral health–related performance and therefore could readily identify the high-performing hospitals. As Chris's team analyzed the data and incorporated subjective information, such as what they knew from visits to many hospitals, they had a key insight: the best-performing hospitals were the ones that had carefully selected their best and most motivated clinicians for key leadership positions, particularly the chief of the Department of Behavioral Health. And, more importantly, high-performing hospitals supported these leaders with competent administrators and ancillary services, such as information technology, facilities, and human resources. While there were some exceptions where difficult problems overwhelmed even the best leadership teams, the highest-performing facilities were almost always led by strong clinical leaders working in stable and predictable environments that allowed them to receive and interpret data from within their own organizations, understand the key processes involved, devise solutions that resulted in better outcomes, and implement changes. In these hospitals, a positive culture prevailed.

Chris's team began to think differently about its role in improving care at low-performing hospitals like the one described above. Team members realized they needed to create stability so local leaders could build a positive culture with their clinical teams. That meant addressing problems, especially administrative ones, they had previously expected leaders at the hospital level to resolve. In the case of the installation described above, leaders weren't leading effectively—but not because they weren't good leaders. They were, but administrative problems in key areas such as personnel, resources, and facilities, along with a paralyzing aversion to any risk, created so much unpredictability that the culture wouldn't tolerate even potentially positive changes coming from the local leaders.

The Link between Leadership and Learning

Figure 8.1 (first presented in chapter 1 as figure 1.1) is a schematic of a learning health system. Two concepts in the figure, "culture" and "leadership," are inexorably linked and critically important to building a learning health care system.

Without a doubt, it takes good leadership to create a culture open to learning and improving. Developing leaders is a difficult task, though, and there is little published material available to guide behavioral health care systems in the endeavor. When training leaders, organizations often focus on creating a new leadership "style" among the individuals in leadership roles. They identify some qualities these leaders ought to have and then set out to create or amplify them in those people—typically with the objective of changing how they work to make them more *transformational.* Two exemplary organizations are Moving Health Care Upstream and Georgetown University's Institute for Transformational Leadership.[1]

On its surface, the idea makes sense. If you want to transform your behavioral health system, you need to have transformational leaders to do it. Several studies have asserted that leaders with "transformational" attributes (charismatic,

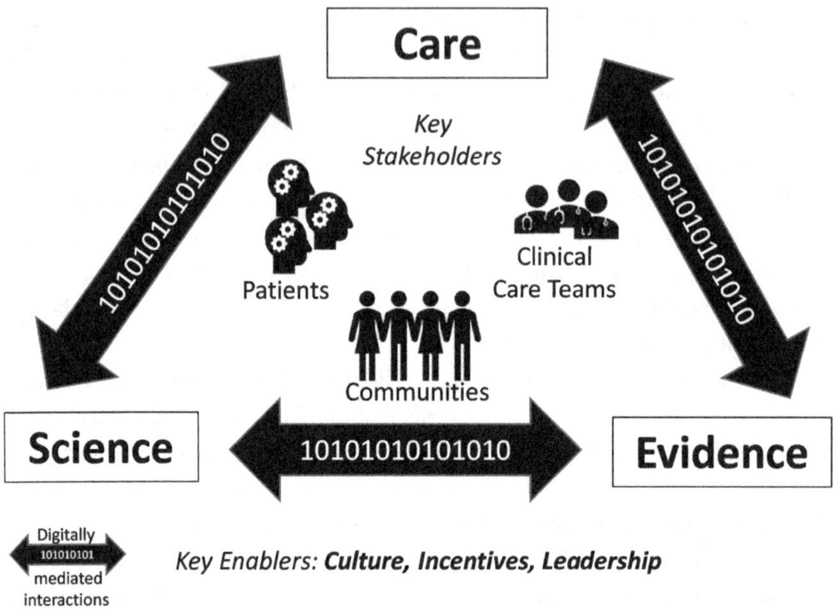

FIGURE 8.1. Learning health care system. Adapted from Institute of Medicine, *Best Care at Lower Cost*.

inspirational, considerate of the strengths of others) increase the propensity for providers to implement emerging research findings into practice, which is a key aspect of a learning health care system.[2] Transformational leadership has also been associated with enabling behavioral health organizations to endure system reforms, another relevant comparison.[3] Researchers have established a connection between transformational leadership qualities, an "empowering" workplace climate, and the willingness of clinicians to implement evidence-based practices in behavioral health clinics.[4] So the solution to the leadership challenge seems clear: find the most "transformational" leaders (or retrain existing ones to be more "transformational") so they can create the change necessary to transform and improve the system.

However, as Chris's team grappled with the problem of improving leadership in behavioral health clinics, they realized there would be huge challenges to putting leaders with "transformational" qualities in key positions across the Army. First, they didn't know of any way to modify the styles of existing leaders in practice, especially in a busy behavioral health system. The idea that a large health care system with hundreds of clinical leaders in dozens of facilities across the world could change each individual's leadership *style* successfully, creating transformational leaders in a timely manner and when lives are at stake, is quite frankly a fantasy.

Further, the Army didn't have a large pool of transformational leaders it could simply pull from and install in leadership positions. The group of behavioral health clinicians that had a desire to take on primarily administrative positions as department chiefs was small. Most providers preferred to remain in full-time clinical work and were glad to leave the headaches of leadership to others. So, system-level leaders in Army behavioral health care determined it would be a fool's errand—impractical and destined to fail—to rely on building or finding enough new leaders of a particular style to lead the departments of behavioral health in each Army hospital.

The Army's alternative approach was to change *the system within which* its local (hospital) leaders worked. The idea underlying this approach was to structure the Army behavioral health care system at all levels to operate in a way that would facilitate a broad group of people being good leaders. In other words: change the system, not the person's leadership style. Solve once, at the system level, the problems that plagued local leaders, so each local leader wouldn't have to try to solve them individually at the local level. Make it easier to lead departments of behavioral health, no matter the leader's style. Of course, it wouldn't succeed in all cases, but it would overcome the impossibility of "training" hundreds of local leaders to become "transformational."

As a first step, the system-level team began to define the essential elements of Army hospitals that were successfully learning, changing, and improving (see table 8.1). Chris's team wanted to know what the best local leaders were doing in their hospitals so the team could better understand what they could do at the system

TABLE 8.1 Essential elements of Army hospitals

ELEMENT	DESCRIPTION	KEY COMPONENTS
Culture of learning	Creates the expectation within the clinical team that to optimize patient care, intentional change is necessary and possible	Stable clinical operations; staff support for change; transparent data
Patient-centeredness	Asserts that the primary reason for any change, and the primary consideration when gauging the impact of that change, is the needs of patients	The patient experience of care is more important than the clinic's performance as described in metrics
Systems approach	Leverages needed resources from any level of the system to solve a problem or overcome an obstacle to positive change	Communication upward to change policy or influence how funds or personnel are distributed; incorporates best practices developed elsewhere in the system to improve local practices

level to help leaders at other hospitals be more successful. They found three common features in those successful locations: a culture of learning; a commitment to keeping the patient at the center of every decision; and a willingness to work with others elsewhere in the system, such as other hospitals or Chris's team at the system or headquarters level.

What Is a Culture of Learning?

An organization's culture, generally speaking, is the set of unwritten rules, conventions, practices, and processes members of the organization follow. The right culture can reinforce helpful attitudes and actions such as teamwork, openness to new information, and frank communication, and conversely discourage unhelpful attitudes and actions.

A *culture of learning* encourages members to critically examine how they deliver care and make changes to improve it. It is the core value of a learning behavioral health system because it facilitates honest engagement between team members, typically using data or metrics. Shortfalls in performance are not seen as personal shortcomings, but rather as signals of problems to solve. A culture of learning enables leaders to make themselves vulnerable to critiques of their performance, which is a key step in discovering and solving the problems that impede effective care delivery. The first and perhaps most critical problem leaders may face when they set out to establish a learning behavioral health system is the absence of that culture of learning. In those cases, it becomes something that must be built—which means overcoming some commonly encountered obstacles.

One of the most common problems is a lack of stability in personnel, administrative, and support functions, which can severely limit a health care system's or individual facility's ability to change its care delivery processes.[5] It may seem ironic, but a culture of change depends on a solid foundation of predictability. Frequent turnover of front desk staff, for instance, makes it more difficult for clinics to implement even some of the simplest procedures aimed at increasing patient follow-up rates, such as reminder phone calls conducted by those personnel. Lower rates of staff turnover and a positive work climate make it easier to establish a culture of learning, because the stability allows leaders and other to focus on learning and improving, not on hiring new staff or addressing interpersonal issues between the staff. Changing workload expectations, shifting meeting schedules, unpredictable on-call responsibilities, and unclear bonus or incentive structures all detract from the sense of stability required for clinicians to evaluate and improve the services they provide. The Army clinics that were best able to implement new and better processes were usually the ones that best supported their own people.

Another problem can emerge from an unlikely source: the powerful "zero preventable harm" trend aimed at reducing errors sweeping across health care. Its laudable goals to protect patients and improve quality make sense in the context of clinical processes that can be controlled directly by health care teams, such as wrong site surgeries or retained foreign objects. But the mentality it engenders may keep people from even attempting to make changes in clinical situations where they can influence, but not completely control, the outcome. In such cases, they fear negative repercussions—for example, if a patient were to commit suicide after the provider had used a new therapy intended to reduce the risk of suicide. Outcomes in behavioral health care are typically determined by numerous factors, not just the actions of the health care team.

In the mental health context, clinicians may misinterpret "high reliability" to mean that any adverse outcome will be an indication of an error on their part.[6] That can cause providers and leaders to avoid changing processes to avoid blame. A clinician who is appropriately using a new treatment technique he learned in a hospital-sponsored training, but who then has a patient commit suicide, should be able to count on support from leaders at the clinic and hospital levels during the ensuing quality assurance reviews. Otherwise, he and other clinicians will be far less likely to implement any new treatment techniques endorsed by the hospital in the future.

A culture of learning includes the idea that adverse outcomes may still occur in patients with mental illness, even when the best possible care has been provided. Making a change, even one supported by data and endorsed by leaders at other levels of the system, involves risk. Clinicians' willingness to take prudent risks depends on their confidence that their leaders will support them if an adverse event occurs or the change does not have the expected positive impact.

The final common problem that detracts from a culture of learning is that behavioral health leaders often fail to embrace the transparent display and regular use of data within their clinics. There is a long-standing resistance to embracing data, metrics, and analytics in the mental health field, where the practice is more subjective than other medical specialties. The psychologists, social workers, and counselors who make up the majority of providers in most behavioral health settings are not trained to assess laboratory values and other physiological data points. Only a subset of providers have embraced the measurement-based care movement and most still rely on subjective assessments to gauge patient progress. Hence, objective information can be perceived as a threat instead of as an opportunity to gain new insights into performance. Behavioral health providers often reject even the relatively straightforward adoption of scales to quantify and track symptoms of mental health conditions.[7] It's not a surprise, therefore, that these same providers—when placed in leadership roles—struggle to understand how data can inform their decisions and guide change efforts within their clinics. Resistance to data is, by extension, resistance to learning.

Keeping the Patient at the Center

The foundation of a learning behavioral health organization also includes a clear understanding that the patient's well-being is the ultimate organizing principle. Every action must ultimately better enable the clinical team to improve the health and well-being of patients, their families, and the community. This is the "true north" of a learning health care system.[8]

Unfortunately, examples of health care systems straying from that true north abound. It often occurs when an organization changes processes to improve performance on a metric, but loses sight of the actual impact on the patient. For instance, there was intense scrutiny in 2014 after it was alleged that employees in some Veterans Administration facilities had created "secret" waiting lists to minimize the appearance of delays in delivering care.[9] While that improved wait-time "performance," it hid staffing and other problems that caused the delays in access to care.

Even a good system like the VA can run into problems. Overall, the VA's performance delivering mental health care is above average, but this episode highlights how the drive to improve services can be derailed when some members of an organization lose sight of the patients' best interests.[10]

Learning from Others in the System

The final foundational leadership principle is a clear appreciation for working across multiple levels of a system. When visiting high-performing hospitals, Chris's team would often notice that those locations communicated frequently with other hospitals around the military and, in some cases, civilian health systems. The staff was also most likely to participate in training sessions and other meetings put on by Chris's team at the system level. High performers usually reached out when problems arose locally.

Learning behavioral health systems are organized so problems that cannot be solved at a local level—be they resourcing, staffing policy, or whatever—can be solved at higher levels through system changes by those higher up the organizational chart. System-level leaders can analyze data to make better decisions, change policies when needed, and procure resources on a much larger scale than can clinic or hospital level leaders, and they do so based on regular open discussions about barriers to clinic-level performance with hospital-level leaders.

High performers also regularly engaged people across their own hospitals outside of their own departments, such as information technology teams, facility and maintenance staff, and resource managers. Chris's team often visited local hospitals and typically invited those nonbehavioral health teams to several of the meetings. When the IT, facilities, and resource management people had to introduce themselves to the behavioral health leaders from the same hospital, Chris's team knew there was a problem. Conversely, at high-performing hospitals, the behavioral health leaders were already on a first-name basis with their IT, facility, and resource managers because they had worked together to solve problems. Learning systems depend on leaders at all levels who understand the importance of working across and up and down the various levels within the system.

Stabilizing before Learning

In many Army hospitals, conditions were simply too chaotic to support a culture of learning—as system leaders quickly realized.[11] Clinical staff needed certainty and predictability if the culture was ever to change—a precondition to building a learning system. But local leaders could only do so much.

System-level leaders realized that to help raise the performance of struggling hospitals, they needed to standardize more parts of the system. So, the system-level team went to work developing standard solutions that included guidance about changes to clinical practice and all associated administrative areas, such as personnel, facilities, and resources, and communicating them to the field. One solution was Embedded Behavioral Health—the Army's uniform approach for delivering outpatient behavioral health care to soldiers in units that deploy into combat. The guidance focused local leaders on the specific composition of all clinical teams: three psychologists, three clinical social workers, two front desk clerks, a care coordinator, a psychiatrist, and a licensed practical nurse.[12] Embedded Behavioral Health required a certain size and configuration for its physical clinic structure. Accordingly, administrators were able to redirect time they were spending to support other approaches for soldier behavioral health clinics and focus on developing infrastructure for Embedded Behavioral Health clinics.

Systems leaders worked with local leaders to identify the programs that should be put in place in each hospital.[13] They also developed standard position descriptions and workload requirements so providers across the Army would have the same job objectives and the same expectations for how many patients to see each week, and would be paid on the same scale. Specific training programs were developed, which added to providers' understanding of the job they were being asked to perform. Clinical programs standardized across the Army allowed hospital leaders to inform nonmedical leaders, such as the brigade commander in the example at the beginning of this chapter, of how the behavioral health teams would provide care to soldiers. They could do so with more confidence because other hospitals were providing the same services to the units on other installations.

Other areas of behavioral health care, such as clinics for children and adolescents, intensive outpatient programs, and inpatient wards, were similarly standardized—which helped local leaders establish the stable clinic operations so key to a learning culture. Clinical program managers and administrative experts from Chris's system-level team reinforced these programs in meetings and with phone calls and visits to numerous Army hospitals.

In addition to a sound foundation of clinical operations, a learning culture in Army behavioral health care also depended on providers' willingness to change components of their practice to incorporate more effective or efficient practices being developed through research, in other health care systems or in other areas of the Army's system. Unfortunately, many providers were reluctant to make these sorts of changes because they believed the Army medical system would blame them if anything went wrong.

That is exactly what happened after the Madigan Army Medical Center, located on Joint Base Lewis-McChord near Tacoma, Washington, set up a new clinic to evaluate soldiers who were being considered for medical retirement. These soldiers had a variety of behavioral health conditions, including PTSD, and had not responded to treatment, and their conditions were severe enough to interfere with their ability to serve in the Army. Part of the evaluation process employed "forensic" elements designed to identify soldiers who might be feigning mental illness as a way to get out of the Army.

When several soldiers alleged that the process was overly rigorous and ultimately prevented them from appropriately going through the medical retirement process and receiving financial and health care benefits, local media outlets began to take notice and publicized the names of the providers involved.[14] Those providers were exposed to angry allegations that they were somehow involved in a concerted effort to save the government from having to pay medical retirement benefits to deserving soldiers. Other providers left their jobs with the Army hospital to work elsewhere. Many of those who remained were reluctant to make other changes to clinical programs, concerned they would be personally blamed if things went wrong. Clearly, it was a climate that could not support the changes required to build a learning system.

The Army surgeon general began an extensive review and an Army-wide task force convened to examine the issues. Ultimately, the Army decided to drop the forensic approach and instituted a new clinically based one.[15] The system-level team identified a more effective and less contentious method for evaluating soldiers with medical and behavioral health conditions that may require a referral into the medical retirement system.[16] The Army directed that the new process was to be performed across the entire system and began to retrain providers in the field on its procedures. Any future concerns raised by soldiers or members of the media would be handled by the system-level team—not the local team. Local providers were assured that as long as they followed the new procedures, system-level leaders would accept the risk of future criticism. This step gradually reassured providers at the local level, who began to make other changes to improve care delivery. Over time, it became common to accept risk at the system level as a way to address the aversion to change at the local level.

Another example of how the Army took steps to build a learning culture had to do with resistance to using data to inform clinical practice. Learning cultures depend on clinicians' willingness to consider objective information about their performance as a valid reason to change their practice. But as described earlier, behavioral health providers in particular are often resistant. They aren't usually trained in its use, and they prefer to rely on subjective findings from their own clinical evaluations. It falls to leaders at each level to prove that objective data such as patient-reported scales and metrics generated at the system level have real value to clinicians looking to help their patients get better as quickly as possible.

The Army developed a strategy to help local leaders establish the acceptability of data within each clinic's culture. Providers had long felt that if the underlying data generated as part of the delivery of care wasn't reliable, metrics and measures based on it wouldn't be reliable either. But system-level leaders had brushed aside local-level concerns about data quality and used the data anyway. Chris's team began to address these concerns, undertaking an extensive effort to improve the quality of the administrative data so the digital imprint of the care delivery process accurately represented actions performed by the clinical teams.

Many providers also complained that some providers' performance on efficiency measures, which involved RVU production (defined in chapter 3), appeared unreasonably high. As the leadership team looked into these concerns, it found significant variation in many providers' interpretation of the coding guidelines, which are the uniform standards for assigning an RVU count to a clinical service established at the national level by the Centers for Medicare and Medicaid Services (CMS) and the American Medical Association.[17] Army hospitals often differed in their interpretations of how to code for things that Army providers did—such as consulting with leaders of combat units and educating soldiers to prevent mental health problems—that were less commonly performed in the civilian settings where most had been trained. The discrepancies further diminished the willingness of Army providers to trust and act on any data produced by the system. So, the system-level team partnered with national and military coding experts to establish a uniform interpretation of CMS rules for all Army hospitals.[18] Several avenues, including those that reached clinicians and coders at the hospital level, were used to communicate the requirement to use the coding manual as the sole source for assigning RVU counts to clinical services. The action enabled local leaders to reassure their providers that workload was being counted much more consistently throughout their own hospitals and at other hospitals. Over time, providers' faith in their performance metrics improved, and they came to view other objective data as similarly reliable.

The work to establish a learning culture continued when system-level leaders began to introduce more data into clinicians' workflow. The most direct example was through the adoption of the Behavioral Health Data Portal (BDHP), the Army's automated method for gathering patient-entered data in the form of standard clinical scales and presenting the results to the provider through a secure web-based portal at every clinical encounter.[19] For the first time, behavioral health clinicians had access to data describing their patients' symptoms at each visit and trended over time. Through BHDP, information on the effectiveness of each provider's treatment was available to all members of the clinical team and was preserved for clinicians who might become involved in future episodes of care, even at other military hospitals. BHDP opened a new era based on transparency and a recognition that the patient's experience of care was a key component of a learning system.

To support local leaders in making this major shift, program managers from the system level conducted training for providers at each Army hospital. They also established at least one provider at each hospital to serve as a "champion" who could be the conduit for concerns from providers to system leaders and for information to be distributed rapidly from the system level to the local level. The BHDP dissemination process provided system-wide support to reinforce local leaders' efforts to shift the local culture from one that exclusively used subjective, provider-centric information into one featuring objective, patient-centric data.

Managing the Learning Process

All health care systems realize that good leadership is critical to building a high-performing health care system, but the dynamism of a learning behavioral health care system demands skills from its leaders that are not taught in most graduate education or residency programs, or even easily acquired over the course of providing patient care. The Army believed clinicians would grow into highly successful leaders of a learning behavioral health care system it the system was committed to supporting that process.

With the conditions to support learning established, leaders are much more likely to be successful in implementing the learning process. Figure 8.2 is a

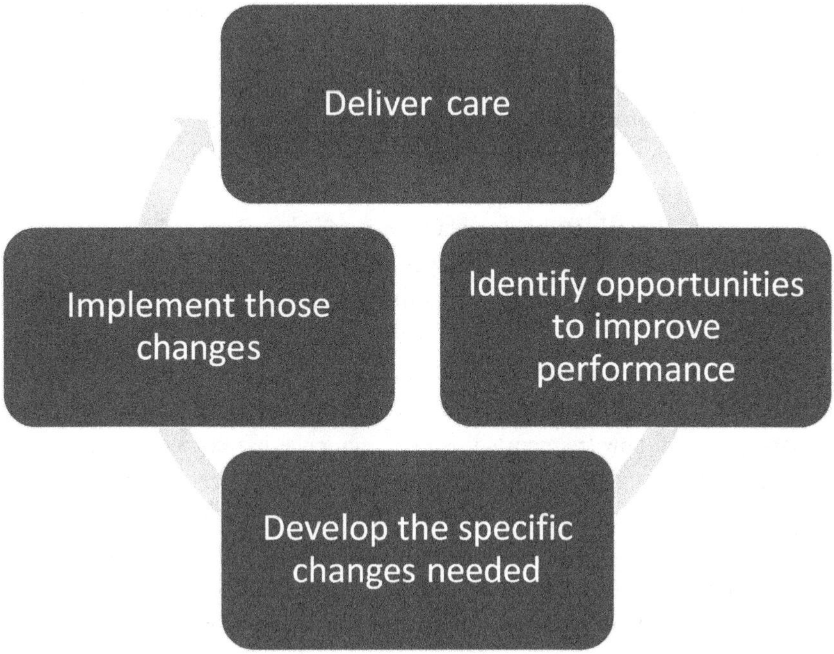

FIGURE 8.2. Continuous cycle of a learning health care system

generic picture of how a leader in the Army behavioral health care system works to ensure continuous learning. It begins with delivering the care itself.

While there are countless tasks required of leaders to lead a clinical team to deliver behavioral health care, two aspects of care delivery in a learning behavioral system are particularly notable. Both were discussed earlier in this chapter: standardization and the measurement of clinical outcomes.

Standardization assists learning because its enables leaders to make apples-to-apples comparisons between facilities serving similar populations. It is also easier and more effective for system-level leaders to organize support, such as training and information technology tools, for a small group of standard clinical programs than for potentially dozens of nonstandard ones. While innovation (in the form of intentional variance) is important for improving care delivery, it is best accomplished on a foundation of standard clinical programs so the impact of a new approach can be most easily measured.

Care delivery within a learning behavioral health system is based on continuous measurement of clinical outcomes, that is, the effect of a treatment on a patient's core systems. Measurement-based care—the systematic administration of symptom rating scales and use of the results to drive clinical decision making—is gradually being adopted across the United States. As of January 2018, the Joint Commission has required use of clinical outcome data.[20] When aggregated, clinical outcome data inform leaders about clinic, hospital, and system trends and is used in combination with other metrics so leaders can take organizations through the second step in the learning process, which is to identify opportunities to improve performance.

In an Army clinical setting, for example, performance on a clinical outcome could be combined with metrics on key processes known to influence outcomes, and further with metrics about the structures required to perform those processes. More specifically, a clinic might merge the percentage of patients with new diagnoses of depression who achieved a clinically significant response or remission with metrics showing how the clinic is getting its patients with depression in for follow-up care or how frequently it is using evidence-based therapies, and then with metrics showing how many case managers have been hired or how many clinicians have completed training on evidence-based treatments. These objective data can be analyzed in combination with subjective information obtained through communication with providers and administrators.

With an idea of the connections between actions and outcomes relevant to local performance, leaders take the third step to develop the changes needed to improve performance. Leaders can find solutions in several places. They may identify the process used by a high- performing group within their own part of the organization. For instance, a given clinic may have all of its providers trained on evidence-based treatments, and the leader has the clinic chief explain the training method they're using. Or leaders may look to other parts of the system at the same level. For instance, a leader at one hospital might notice that data from another hospital suggests a good hiring process for case managers, and so decides to reach out to the chief of the Department of Behavioral Health there to learn how they do it. They may find something up a level that is a best practice they can adopt for their own clinic. The data provide information about performance, but the leader uses the connections created by the system to go beyond the data and find solutions.

Implementing Change

The fourth step in the learning process is for leaders to implement changes in what is done and how it is done. That requires finding effective ways to translate what they find within their own organizations into practical changes that can be made to improve clinical practices.[21] In that regard, it is akin to implementation science, which focuses on bridging the gap between findings generated by the research community and the clinical practice community.[22]

A large body of evidence supports the conclusion that most behavioral health systems do not effectively incorporate emerging best practices.[23] Behavioral health leaders often fall victim to what has been called the "valley of death," in which the challenges of getting research findings into use at the clinical level seem insurmountable.[24] An example concerns the penetration rates of evidence-based treatments in state mental health systems, which has been estimated to be as low as 1 to 3 percent.[25]

Learning behavioral health systems facilitate implementation of new practices because they're structured to help leaders at all levels overcome many of the problems that plague other systems. The close connection between leaders at the system and local levels allow system-level leaders to select for implementation only new practices that meet the most pressing needs of local leaders. While thousands of new research findings are produced each year, only a small fraction are ready for implementation and only a small fraction of those address the needs within a particular system. Implementing new practices draws on a finite pool of time, energy, and money and must be honed to address the most important problems. System leaders have to decide which research findings to pursue for possible application and which to ignore. To make the right decisions, they need to have regular, active communication with leaders at the local level—that is, with the people who see the problems with health care delivery up close.

Learning systems are better positioned to help leaders change how the system works to make the desired action the easy action for their teams to take, a key step in successful implementation.[26] For instance, when implementing measurement-based care, an important process to incorporate patient responses on standard scales into clinical assessments, a clinic in a traditional—that is, *non*learning—behavioral health system might train its providers to complete those scales with patients during their clinical encounters and then enter the information into the medical record. In a learning behavioral health system, leaders at the system level would select a single best method for collecting outcome measures, assemble a team of personnel dedicated to its development and dissemination, and build technical solutions to minimize the tasks required of the clinical staff.

The Army followed this approach when implementing the Behavioral Health Data Portal, its tool for conducting measurement-based care. After identifying BHDP as a best practice that had been developed at one hospital, the Army created a program management office at the system level made up of a small team of information technology experts and clinicians. Their goal was to remove as many hurdles as possible that would prevent a provider at the local level from being able to use BHDP. The program management office took many actions at the system level to improve the patient interface, graphical display of data for providers, and range of scales providers could use, and perfected an associated clinical workflow. As a result, providers in all Army clinics could use BHDP much more easily. They only had to log in to a web-based portal to view the results of the patient survey and could cut and paste those results into the medical record. The program management office also trained clinical teams in all Army hospitals and created directives that mandated hospitals implement BHDP; these were endorsed by system-level executive leaders.

The result of all this was to overcome many hurdles faced by other health care systems when attempting to disseminate a new clinical practice. It was made possible because the Army resolved many problems centrally that would otherwise have had to be solved by local leaders throughout the system. The easier the task, the more likely it is that local leaders will find success in implementing it.

Leaders implement change by monitoring progress during implementation and providing feedback to those conducting the action. Learning behavioral health systems are specifically designed to gather data from the clinical level and provide it to leaders at all levels so they can recognize high performers and address problems in low-performing areas. When implementing BHDP, the Army captured monthly use of the tool in each hospital and made those data available to leaders across the system. The data helped reveal local issues, such as funding or connectivity problems, that needed to be addressed. It also motivated leaders to reach the benchmarks for progress that were required by the directive of the Army surgeon general. Within three years of beginning implementation, the Army reached its goals of having BHDP in every one of its outpatient behavioral health clinics and at least sixty thousand completed patient surveys each month. Leaders were able to implement the Behavioral Health Data Portal because the system worked together to overcome barriers that commonly plague implementation efforts.

The process in figure 8.2 is a repeatable one, which is how the Army ensures the ongoing learning that is at the very core of each local leader's mission. This learning process, which has been implemented across the Army behavioral health care system, involves much more than simply translating research findings into practice. It guides the organization to learn from itself, providing a way to replicate proven best practices across the system and improve performance by using data to help identify what is dragging down the lowest achievers and how the top achievers are accomplishing their successes. Leaders guide their teams to repeat this process over and over.

Selecting and Training Leaders

Learning behavioral health systems use their resources to place the best possible candidates into key leadership positions. In many traditional (nonlearning) organizations, behavioral health leaders are promoted of necessity and lead reluctantly; learning behavioral health systems, by contrast, have processes to look across the entire system for potential leaders

As the Army grasped the importance of great leadership—especially of having a great leader serving in the position of the chief of the Department of Behavioral Health at the hospital level—it developed a selection process to put the best people in those jobs. The process begins when a hospital notifies system-level leaders that the person serving as its chief is expected to vacate the position due to retirement or a planned move, or if the hospital commander (chief executive officer) wishes to make a change due to poor performance. The system-level behavioral health team then works with its consultants, who are senior providers representing their clinical specialties (psychiatry, psychology, clinical social work, and psychiatric nursing). Each of them nominates one to two officers from across the enterprise with the appropriate experience to take on the department chief position. The list of candidates is vetted by the system-level team and the names of the two or three most-qualified candidates are submitted to the commander of the hospital, who conducts interviews and makes a selection.

This selection process drew from potential leaders across the system and involved input from the system-level behavioral health team, but retained for hospital leaders the final say regarding who would become the new chief. Thus it achieved the objective of using the entire system to improve the quality of leaders at the hospital level.

The Army also quickly saw the need to prepare and support its clinical leaders at the local level, particularly the clinicians serving at the hospital level as chiefs of departments of behavioral health and their lead administrators. The system-level team developed an annual training event with a curriculum designed to help attendees succeed in their roles. Table 8.2 indicates the major topics and training objectives. Training focused on implementing standard solutions to practical challenges, not modifying interpersonal qualities of the leaders themselves.

Feedback from attendees has been consistently positive. Local leaders have appreciated the opportunity to meet leaders serving in similar roles in other hospitals, as well as members of the system-level team. They reported that after attending the training they were more likely to reach out to others across the system when facing a challenging problem. The training venue also provided local leaders with the opportunity to provide feedback to systems leaders on policy or program issues. Ultimately, the trainings distilled technical, data-driven work done at the system level into processes that could be used by local leaders to help their clinical teams learn.

As one attendee put it, "As Martin Luther said some five hundred years ago, *ad infantus*—i.e., 'to the source.' Likewise, discussing person to person with [Office of the Surgeon General Behavioral Health Division] program management and

TABLE 8.2 Annual hospital behavioral health leader training

TOPIC AREA	TRAINING OBJECTIVE	INTENDED IMPACT
Priorities of the Army surgeon general (system-level executive leader)	Establish a common understanding of how the executive leader's overall vision for health care applies to behavioral health	Enable department chiefs to develop a vision consistent with the system priorities to guide their departments
Metrics and data	Explain the methodology used to create performance measures; provide instruction on interpreting metrics; demonstrate the use of applications created by analysts at the system level to display administrative information, such as workload and clinical capacity planning	Establish confidence in the information used to determine the efficacy and efficiency of hospital performance; apply information derived from metrics to hospital processes to understand problems better
Clinical programs	Update local leaders on changes to enterprise clinical programs	Improve department chief's ability to manage their staff as they deliver care through the enterprise clinical programs
Resources available at the system level	Ensure local leaders are aware of and can access system-level resources, such as telebehavioral health support	Increase the use of system-level resources to solve problems at the local level

[system-level] leadership at these trainings helps participants see the ways big data can assist service provision, and thus readiness, even for the techno-skeptic behavioral health professionals some of us are."

Leaders and leadership are indispensable in a learning behavioral health system. By creating a positive culture, remaining focused on the patient's best interests, and thinking across different levels of the system, leaders create the foundation for learning to occur. They shepherd their teams through the learning process to perpetuate cycles of data gathering, solution development, and implementation of change. Learning systems set up their leaders for success by supporting them with clear and reliable information, tools, processes, and resources. Leaders at all levels play critical roles in improving behavioral health care for patients across the system.

Chapter 9

TRANSLATING LEARNING FROM THE ARMY

A 2014 special report in *USA Today* characterized the civilian mental health system in the United States as "drowning from neglect."[1] The National Institute of Mental Health estimates that nearly one in five adults in the United States lives with a mental illness, but in 2017 only 14.8 million out of the estimated 46.6 million adults with mental illness received treatment in the past year.[2] The Army's situation in 2010 was similar. The sizeable demand for mental health care from soldiers and family members was not met frequently enough. The challenges did not arise from neglect but rather from the absence of a learning mental health care system.

Just as things have changed in the Army, so too are they changing in the civilian world. Mental health parity clauses within the Affordable Care Act (ACA) require all new health insurance policies to cover mental health and substance abuse care.[3] This has created additional urgency within health systems to change the way behavioral health care is organized, financed, and managed—which represents an opportunity for health systems to meet the needs of a significant number of adults who have not received mental health care.

Increasingly, health systems are recognizing that integrating mental health care into general medical care is necessary to manage the overall cost of care.[4] Approaches that treat mental health conditions separately from other co-occurring medical conditions are slowly being discarded. Separating mental health from other medical care also creates barriers to patient-centered care, a nearly universal goal of all health systems. The Army's implementation of its learning mental health care system can serve as a road map for other health systems, including civilian systems and the Defense Health Agency, which is in the process of taking over care delivery in all Department of Defense hospitals.

Implement Lessons Learned

But where to start? We suggest first defining what is and what is not mental health care by specifying the departments, clinics, personnel, and resources to be included in the changes.

The Army included all psychiatrists, psychologists, clinical social workers, psychiatric nurse practitioners and psychiatric physician assistants in its change efforts, as well as all nursing and support staff working in outpatient mental health clinics and inpatient wards. Social workers performing nonclinical activities such as discharge planning in other service lines such as medicine and surgery were not included, as they did not deliver clinical mental health care. Instances in which mental health providers worked in other clinics to deliver clinical care services were examined and governance established for each case. For instance, behavioral health providers who work in patient-centered medical homes (primary care clinics) are subject to clinical policies developed by behavioral health leaders, while the primary care leaders govern the operation of the primary care clinic as a whole. Staff at all levels should know who is and is not part of what the system considers behavioral health care.

Health systems should then map what they have defined as behavioral health care in its data systems. We recommend beginning with facility- or hospital-level data, using a checklist like that in table 9.1 to summarize the organization of mental health care in a facility. The checklist brings together the information collected in a series of formal operational orders the Army used to collect facility-level data when initiating the transformation effort.

Most of the checklist is self-explanatory, but a few details are important. In 2010, the Army made a strategic decision to separate mental health care and substance use disorder care, which meant that most Army hospitals were required to refer soldiers with substance abuse disorders to another Army organization for evaluation and treatment. This fragmented the care of thousands of soldiers with comorbid mental health and substance abuse disorders, who now had to go to at least two different facilities to receive care. Organizational policies were not in place to manage these patients, which created questions for individual providers. Did a soldier first have to be treated for his substance abuse condition and then for his mental health condition, or could they be treated in parallel? How would the care for the soldier be coordinated? The MIT team used the checklist to understand the scale and scope of care fragmentation at the facility level and

TABLE 9.1 Current state facility summary checklist

Facility name and location

1. High-level organization (circle all that apply):

a. Mental health care is	provided at this MTF	outsourced to ________
b. Substance abuse care is	provided at this MTF	outsourced to ________

2. Levels of care provided (circle all that apply):

a. Residential treatment:	MTF	Outsourced	Both	None
b. Inpatient stabilization:	MTF	Outsourced	Both	None
c. Intensive outpatient treatment:	MTF	Outsourced	Both	None
d. Specialty outpatient care:	MTF	Outsourced	Both	None
e. Integrated behavioral health care:	MTF	Outsourced	Both	None
f. Others (list):	MTF	Outsourced	Both	None

3. Beneficiary categorization:

a. Total number of beneficiaries in the catchment area:

b. Number of enrolled beneficiaries:

c. Beneficiaries currently using mental health or substance abuse care services:

d. Key beneficiary groups (list all):

4. Clinical microsystem characterization:

	Name	Capacity	Funding source
a. Residential treatment programs(s)			
b. Acute inpatient ward			
c. Intensive outpatient clinics(s)			
d. Specialty outpatient clinics(s)			
e. Integrated behavioral health clinic(s)			
f. Others (list)			

5. Workforce characterization:

	Employees	Contractors	Open positions
Psychiatrics			
Psychiatric nurse practitioners			
Clinical psychologists			
Health psychologists			
Licensed clinical social workers			
Licensed mental health counselors			
Licensed substance use care providers			
Other provider types (please list)			
Total number of clinicians			
Care managers			
Psychiatric nurses			
Licensed practical nurses			
Social service assistants			
Others (please list)			
Total number of support staff			

then replicated the analysis at the Army level. In late 2016, after a comprehensive review, the Army reversed the decision to separate mental health care and substance abuse care.[5]

The MIT team found that the greater the proportion of outsourced care, the greater the managerial complexity. On installations without inpatient wards in the Army hospital, the medical team relied on the surrounding civilian medical community to provide inpatient and residential psychiatric services. The team observed that some installations referred more than thirty patients per month to "off-post" inpatient facilities. The period immediately after a psychiatric hospitalization is among the times of highest risk for suicide and other bad outcomes, so when the time for discharge came, Army facilities used extensive case management to initiate outpatient care quickly, often within twenty-four hours of discharge. From a management standpoint, the behavioral health leadership established and sustained deep relationships with its surrounding community to enable the tight coordination of inpatient and outpatient care for military beneficiaries.

As for categorizing beneficiaries, it is worth mentioning—despite how intuitive it may be—that formally describing the patient population in this way is the first step to understanding the known and potential demand for mental health care. The Department of Defense had a policy on access to care that established a clear prioritization across different beneficiary categories, with active-duty service members having priority in military treatment facilities over family members.[6] From a practical standpoint, this meant that in many Army facilities, most care for family members had to be outsourced to civilian facilities. A basic mapping of beneficiary groups also helps identify these kinds of inequities in the system, whether they are by design (as in the DoD case) or are an unplanned outcome of system growth.

Workforce characterization is also crucial, and a staffing summary of the sort in table 9.1 helps identify current gaps and potential challenges in filling those gaps in specific staff categories. For instance, a known challenge in the Army is filling open child and adolescent psychiatrist positions, and the current state template can be modified to capture specific provider or support staff categories relevant to a given facility. The staffing summary also specifically included data related to nurses, because nursing staffing in most health care systems (including the Army) is managed by the nursing department and not a clinical service line. Without clear coordination, a psychiatric nurse critical for inpatient psychiatric care may be reassigned to a nonpsychiatric inpatient unit, leaving the psychiatric unit understaffed.

Finally, there is the matter of capturing information about clinical microsystems. It is important to recognize that the same clinical microsystem may be implemented in different ways. Most health systems have a mix of core (from the health system's annual budget) and supplemental (such as a pilot by the health system, or as part of research and practice improvement projects by an external agency) funding. When parts of a clinical microsystem or the entire clinic is funded by an external agency, the health system either has to allocate new funds to sustain the effort or manage the expectations of patients as the program is phased out. This was the case at one Army post, where supplemental funds were used to create a new clinical microsystem in which providers were aligned to units and spent a majority of their time doing "therapy by walking around" in an attempt to increase resilience and prevent mental health problems. When the program failed to produce positive outcomes, the Army standardized to the EBH model, which placed greater emphasis on evidence-based treatment. The resilience-only program was ended and the staff retrained to work in EBH clinics. The behavioral health leaders on the post explained to commanders the rationale for the change and introduced them to their aligned EBH providers, who would perform some of the same functions and several others. Leaders also educated soldiers to use their new EBH clinics to receive care when needed. There providers delivered a wider range of outpatient services than in the previous model.

Document the Digital Infrastructure

The data for completing a checklist like that in table 9.1 comes from interviews with key stakeholders across the facility, including clinicians, support staff, administrators, and microsystem leaders, as well as from a facility's digital infrastructure. It is important to point out that a lot of Army facilities lacked the trusted digital infrastructure to complete the checklist automatically, and it was only when the manually collected data were compared with the digital imprint that the differences became obvious.

To capture and store the vast volume of data health care systems maintain on their personnel and beneficiaries, health care systems often rely on digital infrastructures that have been cobbled together. Often, there is variation from one facility to the next within the same health care system—which is not surprising, given how many information technology products are available for health care systems to use. For instance, just in the category of electronic health records, the US government's Certified Health IT Product List includes more than five hundred health IT modules.[7]

Health systems must map their digital infrastructure at the facility level to know what data are collected as part of mental health care. The digital infrastructure

TABLE 9.2 Digital infrastructure checklist

FACILITY NAME AND LOCATION

1. Clinical care:

a. Outpatient mental health care is documented using (name of system(s)):

Is the same system used for documenting other outpatient medical care? Yes / No

b. Outpatient substance abuse care is documented using (name of system(s)):

Is the same system used for documenting other outpatient medical care? Yes / No

c. Mental health care provided in the emergency department is documented using (name of system(s)):

Is the same system used for documenting other medical care provided in the emergency department? Yes / No

d. Inpatient mental health care is documented using (name of system(s)):

Is the same system used for documenting other inpatient medical care: Yes/ No

e. Mental health care documentation from other systems is received using (select all modes used)

Electronic health information exchanges fax paper records

f. Substance abuse care documentation from other systems is received using (select all modes used)

Electronic health information exchanges fax paper records

g. Patient-reported outcome data are systematically collected using (name of system(s)):

If there is NO systematic collection of patient-reported outcomes, are providers manually collecting data? Yes/No

h. Clinical decision support tools used here include (list all systems used as part of clinical care):

2. Administration:

a. Patient registration activities are carried out using (name of system(s)):

b. Patient appointments are made and tracked using (name of system(s)):

c. Credentials and privileges are managed using (name of system(s)):

d. Personnel data are collected and captured using (name of system(s)):

3. Financial management:

a. Managerial accounting is carried out using (name of system(s)):

b. Revenue cycle management is carried out using (name of system(s)):

checklist shown in table 9.2 captures the name and location of the facility and focuses on three areas: clinical care, administration, and financial management.

Knowing how clinical data are captured and stored is a critical first step. Army providers delivering outpatient care had long complained that they did not have sufficient information about what happened to their patients during an inpatient psychiatric stay, even when it was in an Army facility! Completing the digital infrastructure checklist provided further evidence to support their complaints—inpatient care notes were stored in a different electronic health record (EHR) than outpatient care, and not all outpatient providers had access to the inpatient care system. Even though the Army could not fix the problem of two EHRs then, a new psychiatric discharge process was created in which a standardized discharge summary document was printed for the patient with essential information on treatment provided and medications prescribed to enable continued care. The same standard was also required of civilian facilities that provided inpatient psychiatric care for soldiers and family members. Although the number of patients who move from outpatient care to inpatient care is small, they are the most acute patients, and their care needs to be coordinated more effectively.

Health systems in which mental health care services are provided by a different organization (i.e., they rely on a mental health carve-out plan) have to assess the effectiveness of electronic mental health data exchange. This assessment has to cover all key data elements such as diagnoses, treatment plans, medication lists, and progress notes that are necessary for coordinating care transitions.

Prior to its transformation, the Army had no systematic way of assessing whether patients were actually getting better after receiving treatment for a mental health condition. The completed digital infrastructure templates showed that a majority of facilities relied on individual providers using paper-based surveys to collect outcome data, but even those data were not trackable within the EHR. A learning mental health care system needs to have consistent capture and use of patient outcomes to enable learning, so the Army built the Behavioral Health Data Portal introduced in chapter 4. While it added another digital tool, the capability it created—the ability to quantify patient-reported outcome measures—filled a vital need.

Knowing how credentialing and privileging occurs is essential for mental health care systems, many of which still rely on paper-based systems to capture critical information such as demographics, licensing, training, education, experience, and risk management related to malpractice. It increases in importance for large health systems, like the Army's, with multiple facilities across which providers may move.

When the administrative data reflect the actual care provided, managing the financial health of the organization is a lot easier. The Army invested significant time and effort to increase the fidelity of its managerial accounting data so that facilities could accurately report where care was provided, who provided it, and how much it cost the facility to deliver those services. The Army had to redesign its accounting systems to track patient flow and build tools such as the Capacity

Analysis and Reporting Tool (CART, discussed in chapter 5) to address provider productivity.

Map the Flow of Patients

The two checklists (tables 9.1 and 9.2) provide a useful starting point for understanding the flow of patients in a mental health system of care. They can be used to identify the key beneficiary groups that use the system, the clinical microsystems used by those beneficiaries, and the sources of data that help provide an understanding of patient flow. If the digital infrastructure is reliable, the aggregate patient flow for these key beneficiary groups can be easily constructed. In the absence of a reliable digital infrastructure, a representative sample of patients can be followed through the system to construct the actual flow of patients.

The Army used three different approaches for mapping patient flow: mapping the flow of key beneficiary groups; documenting key care transitions; and examining care pathways for specific diseases of interest such as PTSD. The template in table 9.3 combines all three approaches to capture an overall representation of key dimensions of patient flows.

The mapping of the flow of key beneficiary groups made it easy to see the differences in patient flow across the different groups. For example, most people in the beneficiary group called "family members and retirees" enter behavioral health care using a referral from their primary care physician or a provider within their patient-centered medical home. Soldiers, on the other hand, enter behavioral health care through their Embedded Behavioral Health clinic. Their care trajectories are different as well. Family members receive most of their specialty mental health care services in community hospitals, whereas most soldiers stay within their EBH clinics.

Data on the five largest referral sources to a given clinic during a month is a useful starting point as it represents a majority of patients using services at an Army clinic. This may vary for a given clinic, and the clinic chief should modify the template to match the clinic's population. Unlike in the Army, where a clinical microsystem is typically dedicated to a single beneficiary group, civilian facilities should identify the volume of the referrals for a given beneficiary group, which can include walk-in patients, particularly if the clinical microsystem is the first point of contact for mental health care. The template currently captures monthly data, but the time scale can be changed depending on the analytic needs of the health system.

TABLE 9.3 Flow across clinical microsystems mapping template

FACILITY NAME AND LOCATION:

CLINICAL MICROSYSTEM NAME AND IMPLEMENTATION DATE:

1. Beneficiary inflow: Where do beneficiaries come from to use this clinical microsystem implementation?

(example: **600** referrals of **soldiers** every **month** from **primary care**)

i. ______________ referrals of ______________ every ______________ from ______________
(number of referrals) (beneficiary group) (time period) (clinical microsystem/walk-in/self-referred)

ii. ______________ referrals of ______________ every ______________ from ______________
(number of referrals) (beneficiary group) (time period) (clinical microsystem/walk-in/self-referred)

iii. ______________ referrals of ______________ every ______________ from ______________
(number of referrals) (beneficiary group) (time period) (clinical microsystem/walk-in/self-referred)

iv. ______________ referrals of ______________ every ______________ from ______________
(number of referrals) (beneficiary group) (time period) (clinical microsystem/walk-in/self-referred)

v. ______________ referrals of ______________ every ______________ from ______________
(number of referrals) (beneficiary group) (time period) (clinical microsystem/walk-in/self-referred)

2. Beneficiary outflow: Where do beneficiaries go from this clinical microsystem implementation for additional treatment?

(example: **20** referrals of **family members** every **month** from **residential treatment facilities**)

i. ______________ referrals of ______________ every ______________ to ______________
(number of referrals) (beneficiary group) (time period) (clinical microsystem)

ii. ______________ referrals of ______________ every ______________ to ______________
(number of referrals) (beneficiary group) (time period) (clinical microsystem)

iii. ______________ referrals of ______________ every ______________ to ______________
(number of referrals) (beneficiary group) (time period) (clinical microsystem)

iv. ______________ referrals of ______________ every ______________ to ______________
(number of referrals) (beneficiary group) (time period) (clinical microsystem)

v. ______________ referrals of ______________ every ______________ to ______________
(number of referrals) (beneficiary group) (time period) (clinical microsystem)

(*continued*)

TABLE 9.3 (continued)

FACILITY NAME AND LOCATION:

CLINICAL MICROSYSTEM NAME AND IMPLEMENTATION DATE:

3. Transitions of care: Identify the principle transitions of care that must be coordinated by this clinical microsystem implementation to ensure patient safety, care quality and/or the patient experience of care

(example: **18 soldiers** require a follow-up after an **emergency department** visit for a mental health condition in a **week**)

i. ____________ ____________ require a follow-up after receiving care at ____________ in a ________

(number of beneficiaries) (beneficiary group) (clinical microsystem) (time period)

ii. ____________ ____________ require a follow-up after receiving care at ____________ in a ________

(number of beneficiaries) (beneficiary group) (clinical microsystem) (time period)

iii. ____________ ____________ require a follow-up after receiving care at ____________ in a ________

(number of beneficiaries) (beneficiary group) (clinical microsystem) (time period)

iv. ____________ ____________ require a follow-up after receiving care at ____________ in a ________

(number of beneficiaries) (beneficiary group) (clinical microsystem) (time period)

v. ____________ ____________ require a follow-up after receiving care at ____________ in a ________

(number of beneficiaries) (beneficiary group) (clinical microsystem) (time period)

4. Key disorders treated: Identify the key disorders with information on incidence and prevalence that are treated in this clinical microsystem (such as post-traumatic stress spectrum disorders, autism spectrum disorder)

Note: There may be more than one implementation of a clinical microsystem, and the template should be filled out for each implementation.

Data should also be gathered on where beneficiaries are referred from a given clinic. This mapping of patient outflow captures the degree of change in illness acuity and identifies where coordination is needed. Using data structured in a similar way to the table, Army posts were able to make informed choices about prioritizing treatment programs for specific beneficiary groups. For example, one Army post found that ten to twenty soldiers with PTSD a month were being directly admitted to inpatient psychiatric care because that post lacked the ability to provide intensive outpatient care. The volume of admissions and the number of patients with PTSD justified the creation of an intensive outpatient clinic, which now treats between thirty and forty soldiers each month and, for many of them, addresses their clinical conditions without requiring a referral to inpatient care.

As discussed in previous chapters, care transitions pose the greatest risk to patient safety. The Army focused on three key care transitions that represent a change in illness acuity and affect patient safety and quality: follow-up after an emergency department visit, psychiatric inpatient admissions and discharges, and transitions to and from intensive outpatient care. Mapping these key transitions identified areas for improvement and facilitated the development of the desired future state. For example, the Army's transition analysis showed that even though a large number of soldiers were being seen in civilian emergency departments for mental health reasons, most of those soldiers were not admitted to inpatient care and, more importantly, they were not followed up in outpatient care. A health system can modify this template to include other key care transitions of interest.

The Army also mapped care trajectories for specific disorders, including post-traumatic stress disorder (PTSD). A registry identified all patients with either one inpatient diagnosis or two outpatient diagnoses of PTSD. Then for each patient in the registry, care trajectories were constructed that captured all primary care visits, specialty care ambulatory visits, prescriptions, inpatient admissions (both psychiatric and nonpsychiatric), and emergency department visits. The mapping showed that there were pockets of excellence within the Army, but there were no Army-wide care pathways—consistent and common steps for the identification and treatment of PTSD. The Army chose to focus on PTSD because of the urgent need to understand and assess care quality for the signature wounds of the wars in Iraq and Afghanistan. Other health systems may choose to focus on different conditions—for example, a large academic medical center in the greater Boston area has chosen to focus on mapping depression care pathways for three different beneficiary groups: its geriatric patients, adults under sixty-five, and its pediatric patients.

Identify and Select Best Practices

Once the templates are completed at all three levels—overall health system, facility, and clinical microsystem—the mental health system of care becomes easy to see. Together, the completed templates establish a shared and validated baseline for reducing variation. In the Army's case, the current-state analysis identified more than sixty unique clinical programs with overlapping and, in some cases, outright duplication of capabilities. Once the data were collected, it was clear that the Army had multiple instantiations of the same clinical microsystem—even though these were not identified as such, they had unique names, and they did not have shared work practices.

For instance, six different intensive outpatient care clinics were identified as part of the Army's analysis: an intensive PTSD treatment program lasting three weeks; a six-week holistic PTSD program that included yoga and other alternative therapies; a five-week dialectical behavioral therapy program for suicidal soldiers; a combined PTSD and alcohol abuse treatment program for two weeks; a four-week combined PTSD and traumatic brain injury (TBI) program; and a six-week half-day sleep and PTSD program. Did the Army—or any health system, for that matter—really need so many different programs? Was one more effective or efficient than the others? If so, why weren't all Army hospitals using that one?

The Army used a template like that in table 9.4 to capture data on the effectiveness and efficiency of each of the clinical microsystems in its hospitals. The information in the template makes it easier to determine whether a genuine assessment of a program can be made. For instance, if treatments are not evidence-based and outcomes are not collected, it's more difficult to assess the effectiveness of the program. Knowing the number of patients treated in a given period (here, a month) supports analysis of the overall value of the clinic itself (the time period can be adjusted for different degrees of granularity). Understanding the scale of the implementation—here reflected in the number of support staff and clinicians needed—provides an indirect assessment of the cost of sustaining a given clinic. Whether work practices are codified supports subsequent judgments about the ease of scaling the implementation to an entire health system.

Once the data are collected on all clinical microsystems, they become easy to consolidate and compare. Table 9.5 shows the comparison of the six intensive outpatient programs that were introduced earlier. The first program (IOP 1) was evidence-based and collected outcomes, but treated only twenty soldiers a month. The clinic was staffed with ten clinicians (including a psychiatrist, a primary care physician, a neurologist, a neuropsychologist, and even a radiologist) and ten support staff. The clinic had well-documented work practices and produced significant symptom reduction or remission for patients with comorbid PTSD and TBI. However, the program provided access for very few patients and required an extraordinarily large staff to provide the treatment and achieve the outcomes. IOP 2, on the other hand, saw almost sixty soldiers a month with only four providers and three support staff, and it collected data on its clinical effectiveness. The overall value of IOP 1 (defined as the outcome divided by the cost) was mediocre compared to some of the other programs that produced similar outcomes with a much smaller staff.

The Army put together an IOP community of practice by drawing on clinical leaders from each of the hospitals that had an IOP. This group designed a stan-

TABLE 9.4 Flow across clinical microsystem evaluation template

FACILITY NAME AND LOCATION:

CLINICAL MICROSYSTEM NAME AND IMPLEMENTATION DATE:

1. Beneficiary categorization:

Total number of beneficiaries receiving care at this clinic (per month):

Key beneficiary groups (list all) treated in this clinic:

2. Workforce categorization:

	Employees	Contractors	Other categories (list)	Open positions
Total number of providers				
Total number of support staff				

3. Treatment characterization:

Evidence-supported treatments used (list all clinical practice guideline-compliant treatment procedures used).

Other treatments used (list all experimental and nonclinical practice guideline-compliant treatment procedures used).

For long-duration treatment programs, list program duration (in weeks) and cohort size (by beneficiary group).

4. Routine measurement of clinical outcomes: Which of the statements below apply to this clinic?

Patient-reported outcomes (PROs) **are/are not** systematically collected for all eligible patient visits.

Patient-reported outcomes (PROs) **are always/are sometimes/ are not** used by clinicians during a treatment encounter.

Patient-reported outcomes (PROs) **are always/are sometimes/are not** reported as part of practice management.

5. Work practice codification:

Patient appointing processes are codified in (list document name and version).

Patient flows within the clinic are codified in (list document name and version).

Clinician workflows within this clinic are codified in (list document name and version).

Clinician workload standards for this clinic are codified in (list document name and version).

Clinical practice guidelines used in this clinic are codified in (list document name and version).

Other key administrative documents include (list all relevant documents and version numbers).

dardized IOP that incorporated lessons learned from the different programs that included more group treatment modalities (to achieve scale) and achieved similar clinical outcomes. This new IOP was designed with multiple treatment tracks for specific conditions such as PTSD, suicidal behavior, substance misuse, and so on. An Army facility could choose which tracks to implement within the standardized IOP design based on the disease prevalence and population needs at that facility.

TABLE 9.5 Clinical microsystem evaluation

CLINICAL MICROSYSTEM IMPLEMENTATION	PATIENT FLOW (VOLUME/ TIME PERIOD)	PRIMARY CONDITIONS TREATED	WORKFORCE SIZE		TREATMENT		CLINICAL OUTCOMES	CODIFIED WORK PRACTICES
			PROVIDERS	STAFF	EBT	OTHER		
IOP1	Active duty soldiers (20 / 4 weeks)	PTSD TBI	10	10	PE CPT EMDR	CAM	Y	Y
IOP2	Active duty soldiers (60 / 6 weeks; half day)	PTSD Sleep	4	3	CPT		Y	Y
IOP3	Active duty soldiers (30 / 2 weeks)	PTSD SUD	5	4	CPT	CAM	–	–
IOP4	Active duty soldiers (24 / 5 weeks) Family members (6 / 5 weeks)	PTSD Self-harm behaviors	6	2	DBT	CAM	Y	(partial)
IOP5	Active duty soldiers (14 / 3 weeks)	PTSD	2	2	CPT	Equine therapy	–	–
IOP6	Active duty (24 / 6 weeks)	PTSD	4	4	CPT PE	CAM	Y	Y
. . .								

Note: EBT: Evidence-based Treatment; PTSD: Post-traumatic stress disorder; TBI: Traumatic brain injury; SUD: Substance use disorder; PE: Prolonged exposure; CPT: Cognitive processing therapy; EMDR: Eye movement desensitization and reprocessing; DBT: Dialectical behavior therapy; CAM: Complementary and alternative methods (including acupuncture and yoga).

Establishing a current-state baseline also surfaces capability gaps that the health system can fill by looking beyond its own boundaries. For example, the Army recognized that there was a need to make mental health care services more available to and effective for children. The Army saw that providing care in school settings enhanced access and improved outcomes for children in some nonmilitary communities. Even though the idea had not originated within the Army health system, the Army adopted it as a standardized clinical microsystem—School Behavioral Health (introduced in chapter 4).

Use Design Rules to Guide Development of a Standardized System of Care

Once the health system understands the current state and has identified best practices (from within the health system or outside), leadership has to define the desired mental health system of care. The specification of the desired system of care must include the portfolio of mental health care services that are provided by the health system (and those that are not provided), a description of how beneficiaries flow within the system of care, and how effectiveness of the system of care will be evaluated. Leaders have to define rules that will guide their own system design process.

The Army established six design rules:

1. The system of care must be designed around the needs of the patient
2. Patients must have a consistent experience of care, irrespective of geographical location
3. Care provided must be culturally competent
4. Clinical outcomes must be used to assess system effectiveness
5. Care provided must be cost effective
6. The system of care organization must actively reduce and ultimately eliminate stigma associated with mental health care

These rules helped the Army make important choices when designing the behavioral health system of care to be a learning mental health care system. For instance, the Army knew that the old system of care was not designed around the needs of its patients. The system of care was provider-centric—patients came to a centralized treatment facility and received discipline-based care in the Departments of Psychiatry, Psychology, and Social Work. Soldiers and family members complained that the system was not accessible. They had to travel long distances to get to a military treatment facility, and in some cases, they lacked transportation. Even those with cars had to deal with the typical logistical issues associated with seeking care in a hospital, such as finding parking. Once they were able to get to the hospital itself, the next hurdle was to find the right mental health clinic to get care. All in all, a forty-five-minute appointment could use up four or five hours of a patient's day! The "friction of distance" also contributed to stigma: young soldiers who did not have transportation had to ask their leadership to arrange for rides to the hospital, which meant explaining that they had medical appointments. For soldiers, making care patient-centric meant moving it closer to their workplaces, in the form of Embedded Behavioral Health clinics. For family members, it was creating one multidisciplinary clinic dedicated to children, adolescents, and families. Ideally, each clinic would serve as a one-stop shop for the beneficiaries it served, which meant that clinics had to be staffed with multidisciplinary teams that could provide prescribing services, psychotherapy, and case management.

The Army's standardized system of care created standardized care pathways for soldiers and family members. Soldiers, irrespective of location, can now access mental health care more easily because clinics are aligned with units. Similarly, family members receive care in the Child and Family Behavioral clinic. These clinics not only provide a consistent patient experience of care, but all providers are trained to provide culturally competent care that meets the unique needs of a military population.

Measuring the effectiveness of the mental health care system is a critical step when designing a system of care. The Army focused on developing key structure, process, outcome, and population health measures that would demonstrate the effectiveness of its system of care. Simple data such as numbers of providers and clinics built enable a health system to assess whether the structure exists to implement the system of care. Patient volume, access to care, and use of evidence-based treatments are measured and tracked to determine whether the health care system has the care delivery processes in place to achieve improved health outcomes. Key health outcome indicators such as symptom reduction in key diseases in the population and psychiatric readmissions within thirty days can be used to examine patient outcomes at the individual and population levels of analysis.

In many health systems, mental health care has not been well understood, even from a cost-of-care perspective. The Army recognized that transforming the mental health system of care would require more rigorous analysis of the cost of care, and it invested in the analytics needed to quantify and manage costs. Tools such as the Capacity Analysis and Reporting Tool provide insight, backed by data, into provider utilization and productivity, which are the primary drivers of cost in a mental health care system. Once the Army was able to connect the cost of care to improvement in outcomes, it was able to better articulate the value of increasing mental health care services and justify additional investments.

What may be most exceptional about the design rules is that the Army not only recognized the importance of destigmatizing the use of mental health care services *but also* made that an explicit element of system design. As early as 2007, the Department of Defense had reached out to the American Psychological Association seeking expert guidance on reducing stigma for trauma-related conditions and on how to encourage care seeking among soldiers and family members. The Army used the stigma design rule to examine each change to the behavioral health system of care in terms of how it would reduce stigma at every level—institutional, organizational, and individual. At the institutional level, the Army actively worked to show soldiers that it was a recovery-oriented organization, and that a mental health diagnosis would not be career ending. The Army worked with the DoD to remove the requirement that soldiers seeking a security clearance would have to disclose whether they had received mental health treatment for a condition related to their deployment to a war zone. The Army put policies in place that treat mental illnesses the same way as all other medical conditions, and it now uses the same standardized documentation templates to communicate about duty limitations arising from any kind illness, be it mental or medical. Further, the Army now trains providers and gives them time to educate command teams about mental health care and shape the recovery environment for soldiers with mental illness. These initiatives have helped shift the culture from one of care avoidance to one that actively promotes care seeking. Moving care to the point of need through Embedded Behavioral Health was a major initiative to reduce the friction of distance and normalize the use of mental health care.

Build Implementation Capabilities to Close the Gap

Once the ideal mental health system of care is designed, a health system has to build implementation capabilities to close the gap between the current and desired states. Ideally, the system will create an implementation framework that includes:

- A single source of knowledge for standardized clinical microsystems;
- Formal policies to guide implementation efforts;
- Training for providers and support staff in new ways of working;
- Implementation authority invested in one organization;
- Systematic tracking of implementation fidelity; and
- Ways to learn from the implementation efforts.

The Army created a single source of knowledge for the system of care as a whole and for each of the standardized clinical microsystems within the system of care. Each clinical microsystem had standard documents such as the concept of operations and operations manual, which were used to educate providers, administrators, and support staff about the design and management of that clinical microsystem. For example, the Army developed a concept of operations for intensive outpatient programs that articulated that every IOP would have at least three tracks: a *stabilization* track for patients being discharged from inpatient care or in immediate need of a higher level of care; a *resiliency* track focused on mindfulness and strengthening skills; and a *trauma-resolution* track for soldiers dealing with service-related trauma. Individual treatment facilities could add additional treatment tracks based on population needs.

The IOP operations manual provided additional details such as how patients entered an IOP (only by referral from a behavioral health provider or after discharge from inpatient care) and which track they were assigned to (patients enter the trauma-resolution track every six weeks as part of a closed cohort; other tracks can enroll group members weekly).

The Army developed and refined policies to support the implementation of standardized clinical microsystems by defining the scope of the implementation, the timeline for phased implementation, and consistent assessment of implementation fidelity—meaning the degree to which the design has been delivered as intended. For example, when the Army implemented the Behavioral Health Data Portal to standardize the collection and use of clinical outcomes, the behavioral health leadership published five policies over the 2012 to 2017 implementation period. In the first phase of BHDP implementation, between 2012 and 2013, the policy focused on building readiness for change: facilities were required to assess the current state and develop needed infrastructure in terms of tablets, computer kiosks, network connections, and trained providers. In the second phase, between 2013 and 2015, the Army published three policies to routinize the use of BHDP, beginning with rewarding individual military treatment facilities for collecting outcome data and then rewarding facilities for additional details such as treatment technique, disorder treated, and so on. Finally, the policy in phase 3, which began in 2017, focused on the use of outcome data for practice and population health management. This same approach was used for refining policies for all the standardized clinical microsystems.

Provider attrition is one of biggest risks with any change in how clinical care is organized, because providers are required to change their workflows in ways that they are probably not trained in and may not understand. The new behavioral health system of care represented a radically different way of organizing and delivering mental health care in the Army. Providers had to learn to work as part of multidisciplinary teams. They took on nonclinical responsibilities such as engaging with commanders and making occupational assessments. The Army trained its providers in the roles, responsibilities, and expectations of working as part of multidisciplinary teams. Providers were given templates to structure their communication with command teams and coached on ways of meeting their nonclinical responsibilities.

The Army's centralized behavioral health management structure established a systematic approach for tracking progress toward the new system of care. Each clinical microsystem had an implementation owner that worked with individual installations to make sure the clinical microsystem was implemented to the Army's standard. The implementation owners created measures of implementation fidelity, such as sufficient staff, and of appropriate infrastructure, such as clinics constructed.

In the end, each system must sustain any change it makes. Leaders at all levels have a role. From the system level, the Army maintained a regular schedule of the site assistance visits described in chapter 7, in which the program managers went on-site to work with local teams to address challenges and educate new leaders in the hospital who may not be familiar with the behavioral health program, such as a commander or deputy commander. The consistent reporting helps clinic chiefs and installations evaluate their own implementation progress and highlights areas requiring leader attention.

Health systems, whether in the Army or civilian world, must develop dissemination and implementation capabilities to manage and sustain their transformation.

Establish Learning Loops at All Levels

A standardized system of care is a necessary condition for building a learning mental health care system, but it is not sufficient. Health systems have to understand how learning unfolds at the patient-care level, within a clinic, within a hospital, across the health system, and beyond the health system itself.

Learning at the patient-care level occurs as providers enhance clinical skills, engage patients in care, and shape recovery through appropriate interactions with family members and employers. These learning activities have been essential for the Army's success in building a learning mental health system.

To help facilitate learning at the patient-care level, the Army trained providers in the latest evidence-based treatments to ensure they had the skills needed to meet the changing needs of patients effectively—for instance, training all Army providers on evidence-based treatments for PTSD. The Army was struggling with the issue of soldiers dropping out of care, and it wanted to enhance providers' ability to engage patients in their own care. The Army also built clinical decision support tools within the Behavioral Health Data Portal to enable measurement-based care, and it gave providers automated charting capabilities that helped engage patients in their care by showing them their progress. This was also part of facilitating learning at the patient-care level. And last but not least, the Army created time for clinicians by reducing their clinical workloads so that they could learn about and actively shape the environment for recovery.

Clinic-level learning occurs when care teams have shared the situational awareness needed to own care for enrolled patients collectively and improve clinic performance. The Army chose to use multidisciplinary care teams to provide patient-centered care, but that meant developing new approaches for spanning disciplinary boundaries. The Army now trains teams to work in its clinical microsystems; for instance, EBH providers are trained specifically on how to work as part of a multidisciplinary team and engage with command teams. Similarly, providers co-located in schools serving the children of soldiers are trained on how to partner with teachers, employ other school system assets, and work with the behavioral health team in the local Army treatment facility. The Army has designed clinic schedules to include daily, weekly, and monthly meetings for care team members to discuss clinical and operational aspects of care for all their patients. Today, social workers have forums in which they share their insights on complex patients with the psychologists and psychiatrists on the team to improve care collectively for patients.

These meetings allow the clinic leadership to discuss clinic performance so that the team could collectively identify areas for improvement. The Army developed a suite of analytics tools that create transparency in key areas of system performance such as capacity, clinical productivity, and clinical effectiveness. These tools were incorporated into clinic management activities to support clinic-level learning.

Hospital-level learning occurs when a hospital can identify and analyze organizational errors, has the structure to support deliberate experimentation when needed to address those errors, and has the processes to diffuse learning across the different clinics within the hospital. The Army recognized there was no single individual responsible for hospital-level learning. Important information, such as diagnostic trends being detected by psychiatrists in the Department of Psychiatry working in the inpatient ward, were rarely shared with the Department of Psychology, which ran several outpatient clinics. That was changed by creating a single behavioral health department in each hospital. Now, a suite of analytics tools that enable identification and analysis of organizational errors such as excessive lengths of stay or unsafe care transitions supports the department chief.

Monthly performance management meetings allow the behavioral health chief to discuss operational issues that go beyond clinical efficiency to encompass clinical effectiveness.

Health system learning focuses on ensuring the effectiveness of system policies and enabling the diffusion of clinical and operational best practices from one hospital to others. The Army's standardized system of care was developed by communities of practice that identified and incorporated best practices known to improve patient outcomes. Once these best practices were identified, the communities of practice codified them into standardized clinical microsystems through policy documents, implementation handbooks, and performance standards. These communities of practice continue to refine the clinical microsystems by scanning the Army for better practices.

Best practices from other health care organizations are a valuable source of learning—a lesson the Army learned when it adopted the idea of placing behavioral health providers in schools and developed its own school behavioral health program. The program offices for the standard clinical microsystems within the Army are responsible for identifying and incorporating best practices from other organizations. The Behavioral Health Service Line leadership also constantly scans for best practices in the larger civilian community and learns from benchmarking efforts with peer organizations such as the VA.

Grow Your Own Leaders

Transforming into a learning mental health care system often requires significant changes to patient flows, provider workflows, care team organization, and performance management. The degree of change needed to build a learning behavioral health care system demands from leaders skills that are not taught in most graduate education or residency programs, or even easily acquired over the course of providing patient care. In many traditional mental health systems, leaders are often promoted out of necessity and lead reluctantly. Learning behavioral health systems, by contrast, have processes to grow their own leaders. The Army learned the importance of having good leaders to guide the transformation of the system of care.

Early on, to cite only one example, we saw that one installation significantly lagged behind on implementation efforts, so we arranged a site assistance visit. It was clear that the behavioral health chief did not think the transformation was important, had no plan for change, and was not ready for the transformation. He lacked the needed infrastructure—buildings in which to establish distributed clinics, network connectivity, and computing equipment to implement BHDP—and did not trust any of the analytics tools. In effect, the leader was the largest impediment to the transformation—and there was no easy way to replace the leader, because no one else in that installation wanted the job. In the end, the Army had to identify a leader from another installation and move that person.

The Army developed a selection process aimed at putting the best leaders in the role of behavioral health chief—irrespective of whether they were trained as psychiatrists, psychologists, licensed clinical social workers, or psychiatric nurse practitioners. Now, once a hospital identifies an impending vacancy, the Army behavioral health leadership team works with its consultants, the senior providers who are responsible for human capital management within the different behavioral health specialties, to identify one or two leaders from their specialties with the experience to take on the role of department chief. The Army then narrows the list to two or three candidates for the hospital to select from. Once selected, each of these leaders is required to attend a training course on the roles and responsibilities of the chief of behavioral health, in which they are also introduced to the rationale, skills, and management tools needed to run a learning mental health care system.

Of course, the Army enjoys an advantage over civilian health systems in that it can order its officers to move to take leadership positions. But it rarely has to do so, because leadership is now seen as an integral part of career advancement for these officers.

The Army also quickly saw the need to prepare and support its clinical leaders at the local level, particularly when clinicians transition into their first leadership role as a team lead for one of the standard clinical microsystems. The Army developed training courses for these new leaders, with a focus on the clinical microsystems they would be leading.

By creating a positive culture, remaining focused on the patient's best interests, and thinking across different levels of the system, leaders create the foundation for learning to occur. They shepherd their teams through the learning process to perpetuate cycles of data gathering, solution development, and change implementation. Learning systems set up their leaders for success by supporting them with clear and reliable information, tools, processes, and resources.

Change Is a Constant

Every health system must be able to answer four basic questions about itself: What services do we provide? Where are those services provided? Who delivers those services? How do we know if care is effective? The templates in this chapter can help leaders come up with the answers. They can then focus on the more difficult questions: What should we be doing? Can we implement the changes needed to get there? How do we grow our leaders to support the change?

No health system has the luxury of remaining static. The health care ecosystem is always undergoing dramatic change. The mix of patients constantly changes. Providers leave to take other jobs.

The Army is no exception. In 2018, the Army, Navy, and Air Force began to transition the oversight of their hospitals to the Defense Health Agency (DHA). The DHA was created after a series of evaluations and studies over several decades, including a recent high-level task force report that recommended that a single organization at the Department of Defense level could more efficiently deliver health care support services, such as pharmacy, information technology, and medical research.[8] In 2017, Congress expanded DHA's scope of responsibility to include the authority, direction, and control of all hospitals in the DoD.[9] The National Defense Authorization Act for fiscal year 2019 established an upper limit on the transition time to September 30, 2021, after which Army, Navy, and Air Force hospitals will work much more closely within a single military health system run by the DHA.[10] This leaves unanswered questions regarding how the DHA will manage the nearly seven hundred hospitals and ambulatory and dental clinics within the Department of Defense as a whole, all while meeting the law's requirement to eliminate duplication and gain efficiencies.[11]

This transition raises unique challenges for the DHA, which has to merge the distinct systems of care that exist in the Army, Navy, Air Force, and Marine Corps. The Army is complying with the law and transitioning its military treatment facilities, including the Behavioral Health System of Care (BHSOC), to the DHA, but there is no guarantee that the DHA will preserve any part of the BHSOC. Ideally, the DHA will build on the Army's BHSOC and standardize to provide care in a culturally competent, patient-centric manner. The DHA creates new opportunities to apply the structured analysis approach described in this chapter to plan and implement a standardized system of care across the Army, Navy, Air Force, and Marine Corps. (Chapter 10 discusses this in further detail.) Whatever that future holds, the Army experience shows that a large-scale change and standardization is possible in a learning mental health care system.

The Army's experience provides a road map for other health systems to transform into learning mental health care systems. It starts with using data to map and analyze the existing current system of care in terms of patient flows across clinical microsystems. Health system leaders should develop simple design rules, such as the five used by the Army, to select, standardize, and organize the different clinical microsystems to form the desired system of care. Health systems should build implementation capabilities to move them into the desired state. The

Army's experience shows that these implementation capabilities will evolve over time, as the health system needs to be able to learn from implementation efforts to sustain the new system of care.

Learning in a health system is not a singular event that occurs at one level. The health system has to be designed to support learning at the patient-care level, the clinic level, the hospital level, and the health system level. The Army's focus in the two areas of training providers on evidence-based, culturally competent care and systematic collection and use of clinical outcomes to improve clinical care are foundations for learning at the patient-care level that must be established in any mental health system.

The Army enabled clinic-level learning by building in time within team schedules for developing shared understanding of the clinical and operational aspects of care delivered to patients in the clinic. Analytics tools were incorporated into the management of clinics so that all team members could see their impact on capacity, productivity, and patient outcomes. Health systems can develop similar strategies to enable clinic-level learning without compromising quality of care.

The Army developed a trusted digital infrastructure with accurate clinical and administrative data to support decision making at the clinic, hospital, and health system levels of analysis. The hospital and health system learning are now driven by a performance management process that focuses on clinical outcomes and population health, and not solely on capacity and productivity. This is an important shift that all health systems will have to undergo as the emphasis in health care shifts from volume to value.

No system has all the answers. The Army continually looks to other health systems for best practices it can incorporate. As a health system transforms into a learning mental health care system, it develops the ability to self-correct and evolve to meet the clinical care needs of its patients, provide a growth environment for care team members, and remain economically viable in a turbulent health care environment.

Chapter 10

THE PATH AHEAD

Today, the Army has a learning mental health care system that delivers patient-centered care as close to point of need as possible. The system is tailored to the Army culture to promote individual recovery and support the overall Army mission of fighting and winning the nation's wars. The Army invested in creating the key structural enablers for learning: accurate clinical and administrative data, trusted digital infrastructure, analytics-supported decision making, and measurement-based care delivery. It buttressed the structural changes with organizational and cultural change efforts that focused on treating mental health care in the same manner as other medical care, creating policies that supported transformation and reducing the institutional and organizational enablers of stigma associated with mental health care. The Army worked aggressively to address legitimate concerns about the system's capacity, efficiency, and efficacy. Today's Army behavioral health system of care is by no means perfect, but it has the key components needed to improve and evolve continually to meet the changing needs of soldiers, family members, and retirees.

It took the Army more than seven years to design and implement a system of care that meets the Army's unique occupational context, mission, and beneficiary mix. But because Congress directed that each of the armed services transfer the authority, direction, and control of its hospitals to a single organization at the Department of Defense level, the Defense Health Agency (DHA), the Army's behavioral health system of care is entering a high-risk period. In the best-case scenario, the DHA will use the Army's system as a starting point for standardizing mental health care across the DoD. It can even improve the system design by incorporating the best practices used by the Navy and Air Force, such as the clinical process improvement techniques within a "high reliability organization" framework.[1] In the worst-case scenario, DHA consolidation will remove the structure and processes the Army used to create and maintain its learning system of behavioral health care and dramatically reverse the progress the Army has made.

To achieve the former, five key risks need to be actively managed:

1. A resurgence of stigma associated with seeking care
2. The inability to sustain measurement-based care
3. The unintended consequences of standardization
4. A diminishing of culturally competent care at the point of need and
5. A regression to opinion-based decision making rather than evidence-based care

Resurgence of Stigma as a Barrier to Seeking Care

Stigma toward seeking behavioral health care was well known as the Army built its system of behavioral health care. Research on care seeking by members of the military consistently reflected negative attitudes toward treatment, particularly in service members with behavioral health conditions.[2] Stories such as the one about the pink rock with which we opened chapter 1 were common enough to signal a real problem.

Army behavioral health leaders designed components of the system of care specifically to overcome many of the factors that contribute to stigma. For example, through Embedded Behavioral Health, the program that moved teams of behavioral health providers and support staff out of large hospitals and into small clinics near where soldiers live and work, the Army set aside time for providers to work directly with the line (nonmedical) leaders. Those interactions were intended to build a relationship between the provider and the leader, who could shape soldiers' environment to a much greater extent than the provider could accomplish directly. The leader could determine the specific job the soldier was assigned to perform, who the soldier's roommate was in the barracks, the hours the soldier was required to work, and other day-to-day realities that could enhance the chance that the soldier could participate in and benefit from treatment. Most importantly, based largely on their interaction with the behavioral health provider, the leaders would form an opinion of behavioral health care and soldiers that sought it out. Did the leader view as weak or strong those within their ranks who acknowledged that they needed help to deal with the symptoms of a behavioral health condition? The leaders would then communicate that opinion to other soldiers throughout the unit, and in doing so would shape how they viewed the soldiers seeking care and influence how likely they were to do the same themselves if someday they needed it. That is a critical component of stigma.

The Army achieved some measure of success in reducing stigma for soldiers seeking behavioral health care.[3] One study found that soldiers with significant behavioral health conditions such as depression and PTSD were more likely to participate in follow-up care in 2017 than they were in 2013.[4] (It should be noted, though, that most soldiers, like most people in general, do not seek behavioral health care when they experience symptoms.) Numerous senior Army leaders have spoken publicly about the acceptability and even the necessity for soldiers to receive treatment for behavioral health conditions. Several have disclosed their own experiences in seeking care.

In a 2019 forum attended by soldiers and held on an Army installation, Master Sergeant Justin Hanley was among several leaders who discussed their experiences receiving behavioral health care during their careers. Hanley, who worked as part of the US Army Space and Missile Defense Command, discussed his personal struggles and his decision to participate in behavioral health care. Far from it ending his career, Hanley excelled. He maintained a security clearance and was selected to attend the US Army Sergeants Major Academy, a high honor for a select group of senior enlisted soldiers.[5]

Forums such as Master Sergeant Hanley's are examples of the changing Army culture with respect to behavioral health care. In 2008, very few senior leaders, especially those working in highly sensitive areas such as the Space and Missile Defense Command, would have publicly acknowledged their experiences receiving care. In 2019, those events are common. While still incomplete, the cultural change is being driven by the courage of leaders such as Hanley.

Another important factor in the change was the commitment of senior Army medical leaders to support unconventional new practices to overcome stigma. Behavioral health leaders realized that establishing working relationships between junior line leaders and behavioral health providers could help positively shape how those leaders viewed behavioral health care. They would be more likely to support their soldiers seeking care if they knew and trusted the providers. But to form those relationships, providers had to spend time outside the clinic, meeting company commanders and first sergeants and other junior leaders, much like the one who came up with the idea for the pink rock. That required time the provider could otherwise spend delivering treatment for patients and producing RVUs, the traditional process metric used across medicine to measure efficiency of clinical operations. Finance and accounting leaders at the Army medical headquarters agreed that overcoming a key component of stigma was important enough to allow designated providers to deliver fewer RVUs than other providers. They would look for positive outcomes in metrics other than RVUs, such as the rate at which soldiers with serious psychiatric conditions remained engaged in behavioral health care.

The DHA will be asked to make similar decisions. There will be trade-offs between traditional measures of success, such as RVU production, and less conventional ones, such as the rate of service members that seek and remain in necessary outpatient care. The less conventional methods may be required to support learning and change within DHA clinics to address stigma and other barriers to behavioral health care.

The unintentional consequence of the DHA making the wrong decisions could be a resurgence of stigma to levels that the Army transformation has greatly diminished, which would have the effect of putting soldiers at peril.

Inability to Sustain Measurement-Based Care

The Army has grown measurement-based care into a core capability of its behavioral health care system. In earlier chapters, we discussed the importance of the technical foundation in the Behavioral Health Data Portal (BHDP), the digital system used for collecting and automatically reporting outcome data, as well as the organizational changes to administrative and clinical processes that are essential for routinizing measurement-based care.

The Army developed BHDP because the electronic health record lacked the technical ability to support routine collection and automated reporting of standardized mental health outcome data. The new DoD electronic health record also lacks this functionality, although its more advanced modular design offers hope that it can eventually collect, analyze, and display patient-reported outcome measures. In the meantime, it is critical that DoD maintains BHDP. Were BHDP to be taken offline, there would be no systematic way for providers to collect, analyze, and incorporate outcome data into their interactions with patients. Without the ability to support measurement-based care at the scale that's needed, the Army's advancements will atrophy.

Even though BHDP is designated for use across the Department of Defense, the adoption in military hospitals managed by the Army, Navy, Air Force, and DHA has varied significantly. In late 2018, Army hospitals used BDHP to collect patient-reported outcome data in more than 80 percent of all eligible visits by active-duty personnel, but the rates for the other armed services were significantly lower. Asked about the discrepancy, providers in the other services voiced concerns similar to those Army providers had early in their BHDP rollout: the system itself was not reliable; the workflows were not designed to support measurement-based care; there were no consequences for not doing measurement-based care; and, last but not least, providers were worried about being measured. These provider arguments must be addressed directly by the DHA, beginning with ensuring that each hospital it manages has the underlying network capacity and computers to support BHDP *so providers can trust it to be reliable.*

The Army confronted the reliability issue in its own hospitals head-on in 2016. In one Army hospital, providers significantly reduced their BHDP use, complaining that it was frequently offline and negatively affecting their engagement with patients. "I keep waiting for the circle to stop spinning," one Army provider reported, "and I have the soldier seeing the screen with me and getting annoyed." When the BHDP implementation team did a deep dive into the root causes of such delays, it turned out the problem was local: hospitals did not have the network bandwidth needed to support the data flows from providers' computers to the BHDP server. Since then, the Army has made a focused effort to ensure that the networks meet the same high reliability standards as those supporting all other information technology systems. The same must be done for hospitals across all the service branches.

With respect to the workflow argument, the same kinds of focused changes the Army made to the flow of patients in its behavioral health clinics are required throughout the DHA. For example, the Army changed its scheduling system to set the appointment time fifteen minutes before the patient's actual visit with a clinician. This created time for the patient to complete outcome forms within BHDP using a tablet or computer kiosk in the clinic waiting room. Unfortunately, the first policy on appointments published by the DHA did not account for the time needed by patients to report outcomes, which almost guarantees a reduction in face time with providers—who now must wait for patients to complete surveys during the appointment itself. The other work-around to ensure compliance is to use BHDP after the appointment is completed, but then the data are not available for the clinician to use *during* the visit. When data collection eats into face-to-face time with a clinician, or if data are not used during the visit itself, it leads to dissatisfaction among both patients and providers. Measurement-based care can be sustained only through a total system commitment to the data collection and utilization processes.

The providers' observation that there are no consequences for *not* using BHDP reveal just how important it is that the DHA develops a comprehensive monitoring and incentive plan. The Army transformed its performance management system to incentivize and track the use of outcome data. Initially, as a means of getting them to routinize the collection of outcome data, the Army rewarded hospitals when their patients completed surveys. Once a critical mass was reached across the hospitals, the Army revised the performance management system to focus on data quality and to drive practice change efforts.

The adoption metric provides insight only into whether outcome data are being collected, but the data used to develop the metric can also be used to gain a richer understanding of the quality of care. So, the Army developed a new "engagement-in-treatment" metric focused on whether a patient diagnosed with PTSD receives at least four treatment visits within the first ninety days of receiving that diagnosis. This new metric uses BHDP data to determine whether the Army is meeting the standard of care it expects to provide. It also acts as a signal to clinic leaders and providers to prioritize care for soldiers with PTSD. Commanders of hospitals not meeting the quality metric must explain to the Army senior medical leadership why they are not succeeding. That level of accountability will also be required to drive the change across the DHA.

Finally, the Army has already shown how to manage the implementation of measurement-based care actively to address provider concerns about measuring the outcomes of their care. Two aspects of what the Army did are worth highlighting in particular. First, the Army *deliberately* decided not to connect individual provider compensation to patient-reported outcomes. Army providers are expected to use evidence-based treatments and justify when they deviate from recommended treatments. Any lack of improvement in outcomes is treated as a signal that care teams need to reassess and revise treatment plans, rather than a sign that clinicians lack competence. Further, the Army decided to report outcome measures at the clinic or higher levels of analysis to make sure teams were being held accountable for meeting the Army's standards of care. If the DHA keeps provider compensation disconnected from patient-reported outcomes and establishes a clinic-level focus on outcomes improvement, it will help assuage many providers' concerns.

Unintended Consequences of Standardization

The ability of the learning mental health care system the Army has created to deliver a consistent patient experience of care through standardized clinical microsystems is one of its greatest strengths. Collectively, these microsystems create standardized care pathways for soldiers, family members, and retirees to access and use mental health care services. Each clinical microsystem was selected by a team of clinician subject matter experts using a rigorous workgroup process to provide the most effective services at a specific level of care for a defined group of patients.

The Army required all its hospitals to identify the clinical microsystems that they used to deliver care. The standardization process began by grouping the microsystems by their intended purpose, such as providing general outpatient care for soldiers. A work group of senior behavioral health leaders supplemented the list of internal clinical microsystems with an external scan to identify clinical microsystems that were in use in other health systems, creating a robust starting point for standardization. The work group, often with the assistance of program evaluation experts, then compared the efficiency and efficacy of each microsystem and selected a single clinical microsystem to be standardized and implemented across the Army. No such comprehensive cataloguing process has been undertaken across the Navy, Air Force, or Marine Corps.

Since this catalogue of clinical microsystems is the foundation for standardization, it is critical to create a shared understanding of what key terms mean. For a soldier, "Embedded Behavioral Health" refers to the behavioral health clinic located within walking distance of that soldier's workplace and staffed by a multidisciplinary team of psychiatrists, psychologists, therapists, nurses, and support staff drawn from the hospital and from behavioral health personnel assigned to the soldier's unit. In a crisis, soldiers expect to be able to walk into that clinic and receive care immediately. That is not the same for the Air Force, Navy, or Marine Corps. The Navy has "embedded" active-duty providers assigned to a specific ship or submarine squadron who provide both clinical and nonclinical services in the sailor's workplace.[6] Similarly, in the Marine Corps, "embedded" refers to Navy officer providers assigned to a Marine regiment as part of an operational stress control and readiness team.[7] For the Air Force, "Embedded Mental Health" translates into integrated operational support teams.[8] Each of these models is unique and delivers different patient experiences under the embedded mental/behavioral health label. The DHA has to account for these variations prior to standardization so it can actively manage changes to the patient experience of care.

Standardization of administrative processes can also have unintended consequences. Consider the case of the DHA's scheduling standardization efforts requiring all hospitals to open appointment bookings up to 180 days in advance.[9] The Army allows its hospitals to book appointments no more than six weeks in advance, corresponding to the period in which the operational schedule for soldiers is firmly established. Commanders are strongly discouraged from changing the operational schedule during that six-week window, such as by adding a new field exercise that would require soldiers to miss their medical appointments. Under the new DHA guidelines, a soldier can book a behavioral health appointment up to six months in advance. Since soldiers have detailed understanding only of their next six weeks' work schedule, there is likely to be an increase in no-shows and appointment cancellations. This also has the potential to affect care seeking negatively because commanders are notified when their soldiers "no-show" for medical appointments. Such unintended consequences take a standardized patient experience for soldiers and create confusion around how care should be organized and delivered.

Diminishing Culturally Competent Care at the Point of Need

Earlier, we described culturally competent care as care based on an understanding of the social and occupational context for a soldier's behavioral health condition. The Army recognized that providing recovery-oriented culturally competent care at the point of need was critical to building the trust of soldiers and their commanders in the behavioral health system of care. Behavioral health leaders had to demonstrate to commanders that the system of care would enhance behavioral health readiness, and build trust so those commanders would then create an environment of recovery for soldiers who were using behavioral health care services.

To accomplish this, the Army recognized and then addressed key gaps in provider training about how the Army worked. The Army realized that for the civilians, uniformed providers, and contract personnel to succeed at delivering culturally competent care, they must be able to "speak Army." So the Army mandated training to ensure that requirement could be met. Going even further to ensure everyone understood the occupational aspects of a soldier's work, the Army created strategies for formal and informal communication with command teams through which that understanding could be imparted, and developed policies that clearly defined when and how command team communications should occur.

Under the DHA, the Army risks losing this cultural competence edge—unless the DHA commits to training any new providers that will be treating soldiers to provide culturally competent care as described above. Failure to do so will further lead to providers not being able to guide commanders in supporting recovery of their patients. But this is not an issue for the Army alone. The DHA needs to ensure culturally competent care for every member of the armed forces and their families.

The Army focused on enabling *readiness* as central to transforming its behavioral health system. The Army recognized that reducing the "friction of distance" by moving care to the point of need, whether it was Embedded Behavioral Health for soldiers or School Behavioral Health for children, would result in more people getting the care they needed. Soldiers do not have to be away from work for half a day, and children do not need to miss school days to visit a therapist. Both these clinical microsystems enhanced readiness, because soldiers can walk to their appointments from work and hence seek out care before they need to be admitted to inpatient care. EBH also reduces the stigma caused by being away from work for long durations of time to get care. It increases provider understanding of the occupational pressures on soldiers—they know when a unit is getting ready to go to the field, when a unit is deploying, enabling providers to tailor their care to ensure continued participation by soldiers and thereby increasing the probability of recovery.

Reducing the friction of distance is not cheap, but it was important to the Army, so it chose to underwrite the infrastructure and personnel costs of enabling access. For example, to implement the sixty-one EBH clinics in place today, the Army had to use a mix of temporary buildings, refurbish existing buildings, and construct new buildings. New position descriptions were developed and the changes negotiated with the union to allow providers to move out of the hospital and into EBH clinics. As we have pointed out earlier, these clinics are not necessarily efficient in terms of maximizing provider productivity as it has been measured traditionally; rather, they focus on maximizing value by increasing the chances of a soldier's recovery from a behavioral health condition and enhancing the readiness of the unit to perform its mission.

There are other models across the MHS that also provide culturally competent care at the point of need. For instance, Navy providers in the Operational Stress Control and Readiness (OSCAR) program who are embedded with marine units provide both nonclinical and direct clinical services for marines assigned to those units. These OSCAR providers interact with marines in their workplaces, as opposed to having marines visit their local hospital. Community counseling centers on Marine bases provide clinical counseling services for marines and their families outside of Navy hospitals. The DHA, as part of defining the DoD-wide system of care, must make key decisions about which of these care delivery modalities enhance readiness and retain them.

It remains a challenge for the Army to connect "readiness" as defined in Army regulations to the definition used by the combatant commands and by other service branches. For example, the Army could determine that a soldier is fit to go on a tour of duty in Korea, but IndoPacific Command—which integrates the Army, Navy, Air Force, and Marine Corps—could have policies that say otherwise, keeping that soldier from deploying. This becomes an issue for the DHA, which must now negotiate the various definitions of "readiness" among all the armed services and its combatant commands, which is no small task!

Regressing Back to Opinion-Based Decision Making

One of the most significant advances made in the transformation of the Army behavioral health system of care is that there is now a single source of trusted data that supports decision making at every level: provider, clinic, hospital, and the overall health system. The Army invested significant time and resources to develop that source and to make it possible to use analytics tools that turn those data into knowledge that supports administrative and clinical decision making. With the DHA taking over management of hospitals, there is no guarantee that the structure and interpretation of data currently used by the Army will be preserved. The DHA must develop a trusted source of data that reflects the system of care it will implement, so there is a foundation for data-informed decision making.

Take administrative data as an example. The Army can now use its administrative data to analyze the flow of patients across the system of care with greater accuracy and thus make critical decisions regarding care capacity, provider productivity, care effectiveness, and the cost of care. The Army uses the Distribution Matrix Tool (introduced in chapter 5) to specify the staff composition for each Army treatment facility. Staffing is based on what is required for the set of clinical microsystems authorized at a given hospital.

All this capability is at risk for the Army, beginning with staffing. In congressional testimony in April 2019, Tom McCaffery, principal assistant secretary of defense for health affairs, noted that Congress had directed the Department of Defense to move away from service-specific approaches to create a standardized model for developing medical manpower requirements, but the approach had not yet been finalized.[10] Today, the Army is able to make a clear assessment of the impact on care capacity, continuity, and fragmentation when a provider position is unfilled. The DHA will have to adopt a model from one of the services or develop its own.

Other steps the DHA has taken threaten to undermine what the Army has achieved when it comes to tracking the cost of the care it provides. Today, the Army requires using the same accounting codes for a given clinical microsystem irrespective of geographic location. This enables an accurate calculation of per-member costs down to the clinical microsystem rather than just the population level. It also allows the Army to compare clinical microsystems accurately across geographies. The DHA is adopting the same cost accounting system as the Army, and the other services are in the process of migrating to the same cost accounting system. But if the DHA does not standardize cost accounting codes down to individual clinical microsystems in the same way as the Army, it will be challenging at best for the DHA to get an accurate picture of the cost of care across the services.

Today, the Army is the only service that can examine provider clinical productivity and team effectiveness. The Capacity Analysis and Reporting Tool (introduced in chapter 5) enables the Army to examine clinical productivity against actual performance and provides transparent reporting at the provider, clinic, hospital, and health system levels. Individual providers can evaluate their own performance against peers in the same clinical microsystem to determine whether they are meeting Army standards. Clinic chiefs can augment CART data with reports on patient outcomes for key diseases to identify areas of improvement for their clinics. Leaders at the hospital and health system levels can make decisions on whether they have sufficient capacity to meet the needs of their local population, and whether they are efficiently and effectively meeting those needs. All these decisions are based on actual care delivered and models of expected demands.

The decision making in the Army has shifted from opinion-based decision making to data-informed decision making. The DHA needs to ensure the same capability to make decisions on the same basis, at every level. It remains to be seen how the DHA will develop the suite of analytics tools needed to support that kind of decision making.

The Army's journey to building a learning health care system provides valuable lessons and a road map for the Defense Health Agency and other health systems to build their own learning mental health care systems. The Army's results show that a systematic approach that builds on the foundations of a defined system of care, a trusted source of data, a focus on reducing stigma to seek care, analytics tools to support decision making, implementation capabilities, and well-prepared and well-informed leaders can create learning at all levels and deliver outstanding care.

We began our book with a story, one that illustrates how the old Army behavioral health system was failing *everyone*. Private First Class Smith was forced by his unit leader to carry a large pink rock wherever he went, including to his mental health appointment. His experienced first sergeant was intentionally embarrassing his soldiers and discouraging them from taking advantage of mental health care the Army offered, because the system within which that care was offered failed to provide the unit leader with the information he needed to fulfill his primary responsibility—ensure the "readiness" we describe in chapter 1. That story is part of a broader narrative about how the crisis of expanding need for more and better care—spurred by the wars in Iraq and Afghanistan—came up against a system that was largely incapable of providing the care needed, and the unintended consequences of a leader's urgency to "fix" that system so he could get his job done.

Today, young soldiers have dramatically different experiences when seeking and receiving mental health care in an Army that is rising to the challenge of addressing stigma and providing the kinds of services that help soldiers recover and thrive.

When a young private first class—let's call him Carter—needs mental health care today, he goes to the Embedded Behavioral Health clinic located within walking distance of his barracks and sees the walk-in provider. That provider conducts an initial counseling session, a safety assessment, and does a "warm handoff"—the term for a transfer of care between two members of a health care team—to the provider responsible for the care of Carter's battalion. If the provider determines that the mental health condition limits Carter's ability to function in his job, the provider electronically communicates with his leaders to recommend activities he can and cannot perform while undergoing treatment. The provider has worked primarily with Carter's battalion for the last several years, so she has a pretty clear idea of the demands of the training ahead of an upcoming deployment. This kind of culturally competent, occupationally relevant communication was largely absent in 2010 and is the norm in the Army today.

The Army's behavioral health system is now designed to work with and for both patients and leaders in combat units, which is a major factor in reducing stigma. Consider First Sergeant Ricardo, whose unit is in the process of getting ready to deploy to Afghanistan in six months. Unlike in 2010, when company commanders and unit leaders had no reliable way to know which soldiers would meet the medical standards to deploy, Ricardo already knows that he will be leaving behind three soldiers, one of whom was recently discharged from an inpatient stay and two who require intensive outpatient treatment. In a monthly meeting with medical and behavioral health providers, Ricardo gets aggregated information on the trends the providers see, such as in the number of outpatient visits for common conditions, and HIPAA-compliant feedback on specific soldiers whose conditions create limitations in the occupational setting, such as whether they should have access to weapons.

In 2010, often soldiers arrived in their unit area after being discharged from inpatient care carrying sealed envelopes containing written postdischarge instructions. Leaders such as First Sergeant Ricardo would have to "interpret" medical language and hope they understood what the inpatient care team wanted them to do. Today, Ricardo and the company commander meet with soldiers' providers before they are discharged from inpatient care, and they work together to develop a care plan that maps out what the leaders could do to support a soldier's recovery. This communication between clinical and occupational care maximizes every soldier's chance of recovering and continuing an Army career.

Young soldiers like Private First Class Carter receive a consistent patient experience of care as they move from post to post. When he moves from Fort Riley to Fort Bliss, Carter can be confident that he will receive care in a mental health clinic that is located near where he will live and work and that is specifically dedicated to treating soldiers in *his* unit. He knows the providers in that clinic will understand his unit and, when appropriate, will communicate with his leaders to support his continued recovery.

Carter doesn't see other processes at work behind the scenes, but several things are happening that improve the quality of the care he receives. For example, the data generated when he reports his symptoms through BHDP are collected and analyzed along with hundreds of thousands of similar appointments that occur in Army hospitals every year. The resulting information is used to refine clinicians' understanding of the things they might do differently to make their treatment more effective.

Every mental health visit is a learning opportunity for the clinician, the clinic, the hospital, and the enterprise. When each is connected, a learning behavioral health system can emerge. That is the lesson of the Army's transformation—one that can serve as a powerful example for civilian health systems throughout the country.

Notes

INTRODUCTION

1. MIT Collaborative Initiatives, "Stroke Pathways."

2. US Department of Defense, Task Force on Mental Health, *Achievable Vision*; Tanielian and Jaycox, *Invisible Wounds of War*.

3. It should be noted that the term "soldier" refers to any member of the US Army, regardless of rank.

4. Cohen, March, and Olsen, "Garbage Can Model."

5. US Congress, Senate, *Department of Defense Appropriations*.

6. Goldman and Morrissey, "Mental Health Policy."

7. Beronio et al., "Affordable Care Act."

1. ORGANIZED ANARCHY IN ARMY MENTAL HEALTH CARE

1. Institute of Medicine, *Best Care at Lower Cost*.

2. Olsen et al., *Learning Healthcare System*.

3. See https://nam.edu/programs/value-science-driven-health-care/learning-health-system-series/ for the updated list of publications.

4. Marmor and Gill, "Political and Economic Context"; Clement et al., "What Is the Impact?"

5. Kochan et al., *PTSI Final Report*, 9.

6. Baiocchi, *Measuring Army Deployments*.

7. Kochan et al., *PTSI Final Report*, 10–11.

8. US President's Commission on Care for America's Returning Wounded Warriors, *Serve, Support, Simplify*; Rieckhoff, "Dole-Shalala Commission Report."

9. Tanielian and Jaycox, *Invisible Wounds of War*, iii.

10. Office of the Surgeon General, US Army Medical Command, *Mental Health Advisory Team* (2006, 2008, 2009, 2010); Department of Defense, Task Force on Mental Health, *Achievable Vision*.

11. Weinick et al., *Programs Addressing Psychological Health*.

12. Nightingale, Srinivasan, and Glover, "*Applying Lean*."

13. Cohen, March, and Olsen, "Garbage Can Model."

14. Scott, "Network Governance."

15. Deal, "Darnall Preparing."

16. Reza, "Chief Says"; Roberts, "Fort Bliss' Restoration and Resilience Center."

17. Jacobs, "PULHES."

18. Weber and Weber, "Deployment Limiting Mental Health Conditions."

19. US Department of the Army Headquarters, "Vice Chief of Staff of the Army."

20. DiBenigno, "Anchored Personalization."

21. US Department of the Army, *Army Health Promotion Risk Reduction Suicide Prevention Report 2010*; US Department of the Army, *Army 2020: Generating Health*.

22. The Department of Defense created the National Intrepid Center of Excellence (NICoE) to help address the growing need for care, research, and education associated with traumatic brain injury and other psychological health concerns associated with service

in Iraq and Afghanistan. Funding has come through the Intrepid Fallen Heroes Fund established by the Fisher Family Charities and its Intrepid Relief Fund.

23. Porter, "Army Comprehensive Behavioral Health System."

24. A "microsystem" is what health care professionals typically call a system organized to treat a specific set of conditions; multiple microsystems make up a larger, overall system of care.

25. Office of the Surgeon General, US Army Medical Command, *MEDCOM MTF Enrollment.*

26. Hoge et al., "Mental Disorders"; Hoge et al., "Mental Health Problems."

27. Standard Form 86 is the form used throughout the US government to collect information needed for background investigations and evaluations of individuals under consideration for security clearances.

28. Soldiers who are administratively separated from the Army have their discharges characterized as Honorable (making them eligible for the full array of earned veterans' benefits), General, Under Honorable Conditions (eligible for most earned veterans' benefits, except educational benefits), or Other Than Honorable (which makes most veterans' benefits unavailable).

29. Army Task Force on Behavioral Health, *Corrective Action Plan.*

30. Adler and Castro, "Occupational Mental Health Model."

31. Beck, Steer, and Brown, *Manual for the Beck Depression Inventory*; Spitzer et al., "Validation and Utility."

2. A BRIEF AND INCOMPLETE HISTORY OF US ARMY MENTAL HEALTH CARE

1. Da Costa, "On Irritable Heart."

2. Office of the Surgeon General, US Army Medical Command, "War Psychiatry," 5.

3. Salmon and Fenton, *In the American Expeditionary Forces.*

4. Hanson, *Combat Psychiatry*, 33.

5. US Department of the Army, *Leader's Manual for Combat Stress Control*, 22–51.

6. Glass, "Army Psychiatry before World War II," 8–9.

7. Menninger, *Psychiatrist for a Troubled World*, 535–37.

8. Shephard, *War of Nerves*, 343.

9. Hoge et al., "Combat Duty in Iraq and Afghanistan"; Vedantam, "Political Debate on Stress Disorder"; Milliken et al., "Longitudinal Assessment."

10. Smith, "Fort Carson Murder Spree."

11. Office of the Surgeon General, US Medical Command, *Investigation of Homicides at Fort Carson.*

12. Millikan et al., "Epidemiologic Investigation." See also Philipps, *Lethal Warriors.*

13. Smith, "Fort Carson Murder Spree."

14. Sontag and Alvarezjan, "Iraq Veterans."

15. Sontag and Alvarezjan, "Iraq Veterans."

16. Hoge et al., "Combat Duty in Iraq and Afghanistan."

17. Tanielian and Jaycox, *Invisible Wounds of War*, 259, 441.

18. US Government Accountability Office, *Defense Health Care.*

19. Kochan et al., *PTSI Final Report*, 8.

20. Srinivasan, Carroll, and DiBenigno, "US Army," 25.

21. Stahl, "Crisis in Army Psychopharmacology," 677.

22. Prine, "Army's Mental Health Programs."

23. Hoge et al., "PTSD Treatment for Soldiers."

24. US Army Public Health Command, *Surveillance of Suicidal Behavior*, 13.

25. Reza, "Chief Says." See also Gray, "Col. Michael Amaral."

26. Reza, "Chief Says."

27. Institute of Medicine, *Treatment for Posttraumatic Stress Disorder.*

28. Lewis, "New PTSD Program Answers Need."

29. Hospitals use the Relative Value Unit (RVU) measure as a way to compare the resources required to perform various services between departments or within one department. The RVU is calculated by assigning weights to personnel time, level of skill, sophistication of equipment, and other factors required to provide services to patients.

30. McIlvaine, "Chiarelli Says Research Continuing."

31. US Troop Readiness, Veterans' Care, Katrina Recovery, and Iraq Accountability Appropriations Act of 2007, Pub. L. 110-28, May 25, 2007; US Government Accountability Office, *Defense Health: Coordinating Authority Needed*; Hoge et al., "Transformation of Mental Health Care."

3. ORGANIZING A LEARNING HEALTH CARE SYSTEM

1. Office of the Surgeon General, US Army Medical Command, *Army Medicine 2020 Campaign Plan.*

2. Menninger, *Psychiatrist for a Troubled World.*

3. Hoge et al., "Transformation of Mental Healthcare."

4. Porter and Lee, "Strategy That Will Fix Health Care."

5. Jain et al., "Fundamentals of Service Lines."

6. Hammer, "Update on DCOE."

7. Weinick et al., *Programs Addressing Psychological Health.*

8. Srinivasan, DiBenigno, and Carroll, "Transformation of theUS Army Behavioral Health System."

9. Institute of Medicine, *Improving the Quality of Health Care.*

10. Institute of Medicine, *Best Care at Lower Cost.*

4. FIVE LEVELS OF LEARNING

1. Institute of Medicine, *Best Care at Lower Cost.*

2. Friedman et al., "Science of Learning Health Systems."

3. Friedman et al., "Toward a Science of Learning Systems."

4. The Joint Commission, *Ambulatory Care Program.*

5. Homeyer and Sweeney, *Sandtray Therapy.*

6. Institute of Medicine, *Patients Charting the Course.*

7. Hoge et al., "PTSD Treatment for Soldiers."

8. The Health Insurance Portability and Accountability Act of 1996 HIPAA provides data privacy and security provisions for safeguarding the medical information of patients in the United States.

9. US Department of Defense, *Mental Health Evaluations.*

10. Malish, Arnett, and Place, "Returning to Duty."

11. The Joint Commission is the accreditation organization for more than twenty-one thousand nonmilitaryUS health care organizations. Most US state governments, for example, require Joint Commission accreditation as a condition for licensure for the receipt of reimbursements from Medicare and Medicaid.

12. Edmondson and Lei, "Psychological Safety."

13. Edmondson, "Psychological Safety and Learning Behavior," 354.

14. Von Hippel and Krogh, "CROSSROADS"; Tucker and Edmondson, "Why Hospitals Don't Learn."

15. Goodman et al., "Organizational Errors."

16. Cannon and Edmondson, "Failing to Learn."

17. Lineberry and O'Connor, "Suicide in the US Army."

18. Miller et al., "Dialectical Behavior Therapy Adapted"; Miller et al., *Dialectical Behavior Therapy*; Linehan et al., "Two-Year Randomized Controlled Trial."

19. Insel, "Anatomy of NIMH Funding."

20. Greenberg et al., "Are Patient Expectations Still Relevant"; Meyer et al., "Treatment Expectancies"; Horvath et al., "Alliance in Individual Psychotherapy."

21. Bickman, "Measurement Feedback System"; Morris and Trivedi, "Measurement-Based Care"; Scott and Lewis, "Using Measurement-Based Care."

22. On the biopsychosocial model, see Engel, "Need for a New Medical Model."

23. Swan, Newell, and Nicolini, *Mobilizing Knowledge in Health Care.*

24. Defense Health Board, *Pediatric Health Care Services*, 97.

25. Flaherty, Weist, and Warner, "School-Based Mental Health Services"; Weist et al., "Further Advancing the Field of School Mental Health."

26. Weist, "Expanded School Mental Health Services."

27. Phone and email conversation with the authors, January 24, 2018.

5. BUILDING ANALYTICS CAPABILITIES TO SUPPORT DECISION MAKING

1. US Congress, Senate, *Department of Defense Appropriations.*

2. According to the Health Resources and Services Administration, part of the US Department of Health and Human Services, "A Health Professional Shortage Area (HPSA) is a geographic area, population, or facility with a shortage of primary care, dental, or mental health providers and services" (US Health Resources & Service Administration, "What is Shortage Designation?").

3. Maslach and Jackson, "Patterns of Burnout"; Maslach and Goldberg, "Prevention of Burnout"; Maslach, Schaufeli, and Leiter, "Job Burnout."

4. Office of the Surgeon General, US Army Medical Command, "Memorandum: Guidance."

5. Fortney et al., "Tipping Point for Measurement-Based Care."

6. Ivany et al., "Impact of a Service Line Management Model," 523.

7. Hornbrook, Hurtado, and Johnson, "Health Care Episodes," 164.

8. Mechanic, "Opportunities and Challenges."

9. Hussey et al., "Episode-Based Performance Measurement"; Goodman et al., "Estimating Determinants."

10. Rosen, Aizcorbe, and Cutler, *Comparing Commercial Systems.*

11. MaCurdy et al., *Evaluating the Functionality.*

12. Thomas et al., "Clinician Feedback."

13. Maliwal, *Healthcare Analytics*, 8.

6. MANAGING PERFORMANCE IN A LEARNING BEHAVIORAL HEALTH SYSTEM

1. Lyons et al., "Predicting Readmission"; Joynt and Jha, "Thirty-Day Readmissions"; Kripalani et al., "Reducing Hospital Readmission Rates."

2. Berwick, Nolan, and Whittington, "Triple Aim."

3. On the balanced scorecard (BSC) approach, see Curtright, Stolp-Smith, and Edell, "Strategic Performance Management."

4. Office of the Surgeon General, US Army Medical Command, "Memorandum: Interim MEDCOM Balanced Scorecard."

5. Fortney, Sladek, and Unützer, *Fixing Behavioral Health Care.*

6. Substance Abuse and Mental Health Services Administration, *Metrics and Quality Measures.*

7. Harding et al., "Measurement-Based Care in Psychiatric Practice."

8. Fortney et al., "Tipping Point for Measurement-Based Care"; Kendrick et al., "Routine Use."

9. Batty et al., "Implementing Routine Outcome Measures," 84.

10. Burgess et al., "Achievements in Mental Health Outcome Measurement."

7. CREATING DISSEMINATION AND IMPLEMENTATION CAPABILITIES

1. US Army Public Health Command (Provisional), *Program Consultation.*

2. US Department of the Army Headquarters, "Army Implementation."

3. Cosgrove, "Healthcare Model."

4. Abelson, "Cleveland Clinic Grapples."

5. Gallo et al., "Primary Care Clinicians Evaluate."

6. Zeiss and Karlin, "Integrating Mental Health."

7. Oslin et al., "Screening, Assessment, and Management."

8. Rubenstein et al., "Using Evidence-Based Quality Improvement Methods."

9. Watts et al., "Outcomes of a Quality Improvement Project."

10. Chang et al., "Determinants of Readiness," 357.

11. Veterans Health Administration, *VHA Handbook 1160.01*; Dundon et al., *Primary Care–Mental Health Integration.*

12. Pomerantz et al., "Mental Health Services."

13. US Army Medical Command, "Embedded Behavioral Health Team."

14. Lomas, "Diffusion, Dissemination, and Implementation."

15. Damschroder et al., "Fostering Implementation."

16. Carroll et al., "Conceptual Framework."

8. LEADING A LEARNING SYSTEM

1. Moving Health Care Upstream, https://www.movinghealthcareupstream.org; Institute for Transformational Leadership, https://scs.georgetown.edu/departments/37/institute-for-transformational-leadership/.

2. Aarons, Sommerfeld, and Willging, "Soft Underbelly"; Michaelis, Stegmaier, and Sonntag. "Affective Commitment to Change"; Michaelis, Stegmaier, and Sonntag, "Shedding Light."

3. Aarons et al., "Aligning Leadership."

4. Brimhall et al., "Leadership, Organizational Climate."

5. Thornicroft, Tansella, and Law, "Steps, Challenges and Lessons."

6. Reason, "Human Error."

7. Valenstein et al., "Implementing Standardized Assessments."

8. Berwick, "User's Manual."

9. US Department of Veterans Affairs, Office of the Inspector General, *Audit of Alleged Manipulation*; Fahrenthold, "How the VA Developed."

10. Farmer, Hosek, and Adamson, *Balancing Demand and Supply.*

11. Stahl, "Crisis in Army Psychopharmacology"; Prine, "Army's Mental Health Programs."

12. US Army Medical Command, *Embedded Behavioral Health Operations Manual.*

13. Bernton and Ashton, "Surge in PTSD Cases."

14. Bernton, "Army's New PTSD Guidelines"; Bernton, "Army Doctor at Madigan Suspended."

15. Army Task Force on Behavioral Health, *Corrective Action Plan.*

16. US Army Medical Command, "Medical Evaluation Board."

17. American Medical Association, "Medicare Physician Payment Schedules."

18. US Army Medical Command, *Behavioral Health Business Practice.*

19. Brewin, "Pentagon Directs Defensewide Use."

20. Joint Commission, *Revised Outcome Measures*; Fortney et al., "Tipping Point for Measurement-Based Care."

21. Bohmer, *Designing Care.*

22. Rubenstein and Pugh, "Strategies for Promoting."

23. Fairburn and Patel, "Global Dissemination."

24. Meslin, Blasimme, and Anne Cambon-Thomsen, "Mapping the Translational Science Policy."

25. Bruns et al., "Research, Data, and Evidence-Based Treatment."

26. Halvorson, *Health Care Will Not Reform Itself.*

9. TRANSLATING LEARNING FROM THE ARMY

1. Szabo, "Cost of Not Caring."

2. National Institute of Mental Health, "Mental Illness"; Ahrnsbrak et al., "Key Substance Use."

3. Patient Protection and Affordable Care Act, Pub. L. 111–148 §18001, March 23, 2010.

4. Fullerton et al., "Impact of Medicare ACOs."

5. US Army Medical Command, "Army Substance Use Disorder."

6. US Department of Defense, Assistant Secretary of Defense for Health Affairs, *Tricare Policy for Access to Care.*

7. The Certified Health IT Product List (CHPL) is the list of health IT products that have been certified by the Office of the National Coordinator for Health Information Technology, which is part of the US Department of Health and Human Services. The list is downloadable at https://chpl.healthit.gov/#/resources/download.

8. US Department of Defense, Task Force on Military Health System Governance, *Final Report.*

9. National Defense Authorization Act for Fiscal Year 2017, Pub. L. 114–328 §702, December 23, 2016.

10. John S. McCain National Defense Authorization Act for Fiscal Year 2019, Pub. L. 115–232, August 13, 2018.

11. US Government Accountability Office, *Defense Health Care: DoD Should Demonstrate.*

10. THE PATH AHEAD

1. The high reliability organization (HRO) concept is based on theories regarding how organizations that work with complex and hazardous systems can operate free of errors. Organizations that can successfully avoid catastrophes in any environment where the risk factors and complexity make accidents normal are considered HROs. See Carroll and Rudolph, "Design of High Reliability Organizations."

2. Hoge et al., "Combat Duty in Iraq and Afghanistan"; Kim et al., "Stigma, Negative Attitudes."

3. Quartana et al., "Trends in Mental Health Services."

4. Ivany et al., "Impact of a Service Line Management Model."

5. DeCarlo White, "Senior Military Leaders."

6. Shenbergerhess, "Dolphin Docs."

7. Burger, "Unique Advantages."

8. Bedi, "USAFSAM Readies."

9. Defense Health Agency, "Standard Appointing Processes."

10. US House, Committee on Appropriations, *Defense Health Programs*, https://appropriations.house.gov/events/hearings/defense-health-programs.

Bibliography

Aarons, Gregory A., Mark G. Ehrhart, Lauren R. Farahnak, and Marisa Sklar. "Aligning Leadership across Systems and Organizations to Develop a Strategic Climate for Evidence-Based Practice Implementation." *Annual Review of Public Health* 35, no. 1 (2014): 255–74.

Aarons, Gregory A., David H. Sommerfeld, and Cathleen E. Willging. "The Soft Underbelly of System Change: The Role of Leadership and Organizational Climate in Turnover during Statewide Behavioral Health Reform." *Psychological Services* 8, no. 4 (2011): 269–81.

Abelson, Reed. "Cleveland Clinic Grapples with Changes in Health Care." *New York Times*, March 17, 2015. https://www.nytimes.com/2015/03/18/business/cleveland-clinic-grapples-with-changes-in-health-care.html.

Adler, Amy B., and Carl A. Castro. "An Occupational Mental Health Model for the Military." *Military Behavioral Health* 1, no. 1 (2013): 41–45.

Ahrnsbrak, Rebecca, Jonaki Bose, Sarra L. Hedden, Rachel N. Lipari, and Eunice Park-Lee. *Key Substance Use and Mental Health Indicators in the United States: Results from the 2016 National Survey on Drug Use and Health.* Rockville, MD: Center for Behavioral Health Statistics and Quality, Substance Abuse and Mental Health Services Administration, 2017. https://www.samhsa.gov/data/report/key-substance-use-and-mental-health-indicators-united-states-results-2016-national-survey.

American Medical Association. "Medicare Physician Payment Schedules." 2018. https://www.ama-assn.org/topics/medicare-fee-schedules.

Army Task Force on Behavioral Health. *Corrective Action Plan.* Fort Sam Houston, TX: Department of the Army, 2013.

Baiocchi, Dave. *Measuring Army Deployments to Iraq and Afghanistan.* Santa Monica, CA: RAND Corporation, 2013. https://www.rand.org/pubs/research_reports/RR145.html.

Batty, Martin J., Maria Moldavsky, Pooria Sarrami Foroushani, Sarah Pass, Michael Marriott, Kapil Sayal, and Chris Hollis. "Implementing Routine Outcome Measures in Child and Adolescent Mental Health Services: From Pesent to Future Practice." *Child and Adolescent Mental Health* 18, no. 2 (2013): 82–87.

Beck, Aaron T., Robert A. Steer, and Gregory K. Brown. *Manual for the Beck Depression Inventory–II.* San Antonio, TX: Psychological Corporation, 1996.

Bedi, Shireen. "USAFSAM Readies Operational Mental Health Care Providers." *Air Force Medical Service*, October 18, 2018. https://www.airforcemedicine.af.mil/News/Display/Article/1665939/usafsam-readies-operational-mental-health-care-providers/

Bernton, Hal. "Army Doctor at Madigan Suspended over PTSD Comments." *Seattle Times*, February 3, 2012. https://www.seattletimes.com/seattle-news/army-doctor-at-madigan-suspended-over-ptsd-comments/.

——. "Army's New PTSD Guidelines Fault Madigan's Screening Tests." *Seattle Times*, April 21, 2012. https://www.seattletimes.com/seattle-news/armys-new-ptsd-guidelines-fault-madigans-screening-tests/.

Bernton, Hal, and Adam Ashton. "Surge in PTSD Cases Has Army Overhauling Mental Health Services." *Spokesman-Review* (Spokane, WA), May 17, 2015. http://www.spokesman.com/stories/2015/may/17/surge-in-ptsd-cases-has-army-overhauling-mental/.

Beronio, Kirsten, Sherry Glied, and Richard Frank. "How the Affordable Care Act and Mental Health Parity and Addiction Equity Act Greatly Expand Coverage of Behavioral Health Care." *Journal of Behavioral Health Services and Research* 41, no. 4 (2014): 410–28.

Berwick, Donald M. "A User's Manual for the IOM's 'Quality Chasm' Report." *Health Affairs* 21, no. 3 (2002): 80–90.

Berwick, Donald M., Thomas W. Nolan, and John Whittington. "The Triple Aim: Care, Health, and Cost." *Health Affairs* 27, no. 3 (2008): 759–69.

Bickman, Leonard. "A Measurement Feedback System (MFS) Is Necessary to Improve Mental Health Outcomes." *Journal of the American Academy of Child and Adolescent Psychiatry* 47, no. 10 (2008): 1114–19.

Bohmer, Richard M. J. *Designing Care: Aligning the Nature and Management of Health Care.* Boston: Harvard Business Press, 2009.

Brewin, Bob. "Pentagon Directs Defensewide Use of Army's Mental Health Data Portal." *NextGov*, October 30, 2013. https://www.nextgov.com/it-modernization/2013/10/pentagon-directs-defensewide-use-armys-mental-health-data-portal/72953/.

Brimhall, Kim C., Karissa Fenwick, Lauren R. Farahnak, Michael S. Hurlburt, Scott C. Roesch, and Gregory A. Aarons. "Leadership, Organizational Climate, and Perceived Burden of Evidence-Based Practice in Mental Health Services." *Administration and Policy in Mental Health and Mental Health Services Research* 43, no. 5 (2016): 629–39.

Bruns, Eric J., Suzanne E. U. Kerns, Michael D. Pullmann, Spencer W. Hensley, Ted Lutterman, and Kimberly E. Hoagwood. "Research, Data, and Evidence-Based Treatment Use in State Behavioral Health Systems, 2001–2012." *Psychiatric Services* 67, no. 5 (2016): 496–503.

Burger, John M. "Unique Advantages of Embedded OSCAR Teams." *Navy Medicine Live*, March 25, 2021. https://navymedicine.navylive.dodlive.mil/archives/10422.

Burgess, Philip, Tim Coombs, Adam Clarke, Rosemary Dickson, and Jane Pirkis. "Achievements in Mental Health Outcome Measurement in Australia: Reflections on Progress Made by the Australian Mental Health Outcomes and Classification Network (AMHOCN)." *International Journal of Mental Health Systems* 6, no. 1 (2012): 4.

Cannon, Mark D., and Amy C. Edmondson. "Failing to Learn and Learning to Fail (Intelligently): How Great Organizations Put Failure to Work to Innovate and Improve." *Long Range Planning* 38, no. 3 (2005): 299–319.

Carroll, Christopher, Malcolm Patterson, Stephen Wood, Andrew Booth, Jo Rick, and Shashi Balain. "A Conceptual Framework for Implementation Fidelity." *Implementation Science* 2, no. 1 (2007): 40.

Carroll, J. S., and J. W. Rudolph. "Design of High Reliability Organizations in Health Care." *BMJ Quality & Safety* 15, no. suppl. 1 (2006): i4–i9.

Chang, Evelyn T., Danielle E. Rose, Elizabeth M. Yano, Kenneth B. Wells, Maureen E. Metzger, Edward P. Post, Martin L. Lee, and Lisa V. Rubenstein. "Determinants of Readiness for Primary Care–Mental Health Integration (PC-MHI) in the VA Health Care System." *Journal of General Internal Medicine* 28, no. 3 (2013): 353–62.

Clement, S., O. Schauman, T. Graham, F. Maggioni, S. Evans-Lacko, N. Bezborodovs, C. Morgan, N. Rüsch, J. S. L. Brown, and G. Thornicroft. "What Is the Impact of Mental Health–Related Stigma on Help-Seeking? A Systematic Review of Quantitative and Qualitative Studies." *Psychological Medicine* 45, no. 1 (2015): 11–27.

Cohen, Michael D., James G. March, and Johan P. Olsen. "A Garbage Can Model of Organizational Choice." *Administrative Science Quarterly* 17, no. 1 (1972): 1–25.

Cosgrove, Delos M. "A Healthcare Model for the 21st Century: Patient-Centered, Integrated Delivery System." *Group Practice Journal of the American Medical Group Association* 60, no. 3 (March 2011): 11–15.

Curtright, Jonathan W., Steven C. Stolp-Smith, and Eric S. Edell. "Strategic Performance Management: Development of a Performance Measurement System at the Mayo Clinic." *Journal of Healthcare Management* 45, no. 1 (2000): 58–68.

Da Costa, Jacob M. "ART. I.–On Irritable Heart; a Clinical Study of a Form of Functional Cardiac Disorder and its Consequences." *The American Journal of the Medical Sciences (1827–1924)* 61, no. 121 (1871): 17.

Damschroder, Laura J., David C. Aron, Rosalind E. Keith, Susan R. Kirsh, Jeffery A. Alexander, and Julie C. Lowery. "Fostering Implementation of Health Services Research Findings into Practice: A Consolidated Framework for Advancing Implementation Science." *Implementation Science* 4, no. 1 (2009): 50.

Deal, Patricia. "Darnall Preparing to Meet Growing Demand for Behavioral Health Services for Returning Soldiers." US Army, December 6, 2011. https://www.army.mil/article/70344/darnall_preparing_to_meet_growing_demand_for_behavioral_health_services_for_returning_soldiers.

DeCarloWhite, Holly. "Senior Military Leaders Share Experience in Experiences in Mental Health." US Army, April 22, 2019. https://www.army.mil/article/220665/senior_military_leaders_share_experiences_in_mental_health.

Defense Health Agency. "Standard Appointing Processes, Procedures, Hours of Operation, Productivity, Performance Measures and Appointment Types in Primary, Specialty, and Behavioral Health Care in Medical Treatment Facilities (MTFs)." Interim Procedures Memorandum 18-001. https:/health.mil/Reference-Center/Policies/2020/02/04/DHA-IPM-18-001-Standard-Appointing-Processes-Procedures.

Defense Health Board. *Pediatric Health Care Services.* Falls Church, VA: Defense Health Board, 2017. http://www.tricareforkids.org/wp-content/uploads/2017/08/Pediatric-Health-Care-Services-Report-080717-Predecisional-Draft.pdf.

DiBenigno, Julia. "Anchored Personalization in Managing Goal Conflict between Professional Groups: The Case of U.S. Army Mental Health Care." *Administrative Science Quarterly* 63, no. 3 (2018): 526–69.

Dundon, M., K. Dollar, M. Schohn, and L. J. Lantinga. *Primary Care–Mental Health Integration Co-located, Collaborative Care: An Operations Manual.* Syracuse, NY: VA Center for Integrated Healthcare, 2011.

Edmondson, Amy. "Psychological Safety and Learning Behavior in Work Teams." *Administrative Science Quarterly* 44, no. 2 (1999): 350–83.

Edmondson, Amy C., and Zhike Lei. "Psychological Safety: The History, Renaissance, and Future of an Interpersonal Construct." *Annual Review of Organizational Psychology and Organizational Behavior* 1, no. 1 (2014): 23–43.

Engel, G. L. "The Need for a New Medical Model: A Challenge for Biomedicine." *Science* 196, no. 4286 (1977): 129–36.

Fahrenthold, David. "How the VA Developed Its Culture of Coverups." *Washington Post,* May 30, 2014. http://www.washingtonpost.com/sf/national/2014/05/30/how-the-va-developed-its-culture-of-coverups/.

Fairburn, Christopher G., and Vikram Patel. "The Global Dissemination of Psychological Treatments: A Road Map for Research and Practice." *American Journal of Psychiatry* 171, no. 5 (2014): 495–98.

Farmer, Carrie M., Susan D. Hosek, and David M. Adamson. *Balancing Demand and Supply for Veterans' Health Care: A Summary of Three RAND Assessments Conducted under the Veterans Choice Act*. Santa Monica, CA: RAND Corporation, 2016. https://www.rand.org/pubs/research_reports/RR1165z4.html.

Flaherty, Lois T., Mark D. Weist, and Beth S. Warner. "School-Based Mental Health Services in the United States: History, Current Models and Needs." *Community Mental Health Journal* 32, no. 4 (1996): 341–52.

Fortney, John C., Rebecca Sladek, and Jürgen Unützer. *Fixing Behavioral Healthcare in America: A National Call for Measurement-Based Care in the Delivery of Behavioral Health Services*. Island Heights, NJ: The Kennedy Forum, 2015. https://www.thekennedyforum.org/app/uploads/2017/06/KennedyForum-MeasurementBasedCare_2.pdf.

Fortney, John C., Jürgen Unützer, Glenda Wrenn, Jeffrey M. Pyne, Richard G. Smith, Michael Schoenbaum, and Henry T. Harbin. "A Tipping Point for Measurement-Based Care." *Psychiatric Services* 68, no. 2 (2017): 179–88.

Friedman, Charles P., Nancy J. Allee, Brendan C. Delaney, Allen J. Flynn, Jonathan C. Silverstein, Kevin Sullivan, and Kathleen A. Young. "The Science of Learning Health Systems: Foundations for a New Journal." *Learning Health Systems* 1, no. 1 (2017): e10020.

Friedman, Charles P., Joshua Rubin, Jeffrey Brown, Melinda Buntin, Milton Corn, Lynn Etheredge, Carl Gunter, Mark Musen, Richard Platt, William Stead, Kevin Sullivan, and Douglas Van Houweling. "Toward a Science of Learning Systems: A Research Agenda for the High-Functioning Learning Health System." *Journal of the American Medical Informatics Association* 22, no. 1 (2014): 43–50.

Fullerton, Catherine A., Rachel M. Henke, Erica L. Carable, Andriana Hohlbauch, and Nicholas Cummings. "The Impact of Medicare ACOs on Improving Integration and Coordination of Physical and Behavioral Health Care." *Health Affairs* 35, no. 7 (2016): 1257–65.

Gallo, Joseph J., Cynthia Zubritsky, James Maxwell, Michael Nazar, Hillary R. Bogner, Louise M. Quijano, Heidi J. Syropoulos, Karen L. Cheal, Hongtu Chen, Herman Sanchez, John Dodson, Sue E. Levkoff, and the Prism-E Investigators. "Primary Care Clinicians Evaluate Integrated and Referral Models of Behavioral Health Care for Older Adults: Results from a Multisite Effectiveness Trial (PRISM-E)." *Annals of Family Medicine* 2, no. 4 (2004): 305–9.

Glass, Albert J. "Army Psychiatry before World War II." *Medical Department United States Army. Neuropsychiatry in World War II* 1 (1966): 3–23.

Goldman H. H., and J. P. Morrissey. "Mental Health Policy: Fundamental Reform or Incremental Change?" In *The Palgrave Handbook of American Mental Health Policy*, edited by H. Goldman, R. Frank, and J. Morrissey, 3–20. Cham, Switzerland: Palgrave Macmillan, 2020. https://doi.org/10.1007/978-3-030-11908-9_1.

Goodman, Allen C., Janet R. Hankin, David E. Kalist, Yingwei Peng, and Stephen J. Spurr. "Estimating Determinants of Multiple Treatment Episodes for Substance Abusers." *Journal of Mental Health Policy and Economics* 4, no. 2 (2001): 65–77.

Goodman, Paul S., Rangaraj Ramanujam, John S. Carroll, Amy C. Edmondson, David A. Hofmann, and Kathleen M. Sutcliffe. "Organizational Errors: Directions for Future Research." *Research in Organizational Behavior* 31 (2011): 151–76.

Gray, Robert. "Col. Michael Amaral—Chief of Staff, Beaumont Medical Center: The $1-Billion Challenge." *El Paso Times*, March 19, 2012. http://www.elpasoinc.com/news/q_and_a/col-michael-amaral—chief-of-staff-beaumont-medical-center/article_e4f66a68-71de-11e1-b322-0019bb30f31a.html.

Greenberg, Roger P., Michael J. Constantino, and Noah Bruce. "Are Patient Expectations Still Relevant for Psychotherapy Process and Outcome?" *Clinical Psychology Review* 26, no. 6 (2006): 657–78.

Halvorson, George C. *Health Care Will Not Reform Itself: A User's Guide to Refocusing and Reforming American Health Care.* New York: Productivity Press, 2009.

Hamilton, John D., and Leonard Bickman. "A Measurement Feedback System (MFS) Is Necessary to Improve Mental Health Outcomes." *Journal of the American Academy of Child and Adolescent Psychiatry* 47, no. 10 (2008): 1114–19.

Hammer, Paul. "Update on DCOE." Defense Health Board, March 8, 2011. https://health.mil/Reference-Center/Presentations/2011/03/08/Defense-Centers-of-Excellence-for-Psychological-Health-and-Traumatic-Brain-Injury-Briefing.

Hanson, Frederick, ed. *Combat Psychiatry: Experiences in the North African and Mediterranean Theaters of Operation, American Ground Forces, World War II.* Vol. 9 suppl., *Bulletin of the U.S. Army Medical Department.* Washington, DC: 1949.

Harding, Kelli Jane K., A. John Rush, Melissa Arbuckle, Madhukar H. Trivedi, and Harold Alan Pincus. "Measurement-Based Care in Psychiatric Practice: A Policy Framework for Implementation." *Journal of Clinical Psychiatry* 72, no. 8 (2011): 1136–43.

Hoge, Charles W., Jennifer L. Auchterlonie, and Charles S. Milliken. "Mental Health Problems, Use of Mental Health Services, and Attrition from Military Service after Returning from Deployment to Iraq or Afghanistan." *JAMA* 295, no. 9 (2006): 1023–32.

Hoge, Charles W., Carl A. Castro, Stephen C. Messer, Dennis McGurk, Dave I. Cotting, and Robert L. Koffman. "Combat Duty in Iraq and Afghanistan, Mental Health Problems, and Barriers to Care." *New England Journal of Medicine* 351, no. 1 (2004): 13–22.

Hoge, Charles W., Sasha H. Grossman, Jennifer L. Auchterlonie, Lyndon A. Riviere, Charles S. Milliken, and Joshua E. Wilk. "PTSD Treatment for Soldiers after Combat Deployment: Low Utilization of Mental Health Care and Reasons for Dropout." *Psychiatric Services* 65, no. 8 (2014): 997–1004.

Hoge, Charles W., Christopher G. Ivany, Edward A. Brusher, Millard D. Brown III, John C. Shero, Amy B. Adler, Christopher H. Warner, and David T. Orman. "Transformation of Mental Health Care for U.S. Soldiers and Families during the Iraq and Afghanistan Wars: Where Science and Politics Intersect." *American Journal of Psychiatry* 173, no. 4 (2016): 334–43.

Hoge, Charles W., Sandra E. Lesikar, Ramon Guevara, Jeff Lange, John F. Brundage, Charles C. Engel, Stephen C. Messer, and David T. Orman. "Mental Disorders among U.S. Military Personnel in the 1990s: Association with High Levels of Health Care Utilization and Early Military Attrition." *American Journal of Psychiatry* 159, no. 9 (2002): 1576–83.

Homeyer, Linda E., and Daniel S. Sweeney. *Sandtray Therapy: A Practical Manual.* New York: Routledge, 2016.

Hornbrook, Mark C., Arnold V. Hurtado, and Richard E. Johnson. "Health Care Episodes: Definition, Measurement and Use." *Medical Care Review* 42, no. 2 (1985): 163–218.

Horvath, Adam O., A. C. Del Re, Christoph Flückiger, and Dianne Symonds. "Alliance in Individual Psychotherapy." *Psychotherapy* 48, no. 1 (2011): 9–16.

Hussey, Peter S., Melony E. Sorbero, Ateev Mehrotra, Liu Hangsheng, and Cheryl L. Damberg. "Episode-Based Performance Measurement and Payment: Making It a Reality." *Health Affairs* 28, no. 5 (2009): 1406–17.

Insel, Thomas R. "The Anatomy of NIMH Funding." National Institute of Mental Health, 2015.

———. "Transparency." Blog post. National Institute of Mental Health, 2015. https://www.nimh.nih.gov/about/directors/thomas-insel/blog/2015/transparency.shtml.

Institute of Medicine. *Best Care at Lower Cost: The Path to Continuously Learning Health Care in America*. Edited by Mark Smith, Robert Saunders, Leigh Stuckhardt, and J. Michael McGinnis. Washington, DC: National Academies Press, 2013. doi:10.17226/13444.

——. *Improving the Quality of Health Care for Mental and Substance-Use Conditions*. Washington, DC: National Academies Press, 2006. doi:10.17226/11470.

——. *The Learning Healthcare System: Workshop Summary*. Edited by LeighAnne Olsen, Dara Aisner, and J. Michael McGinnis. Washington, DC: National Academies Press, 2007. doi:10.17226/11903.

——. *Patients Charting the Course: Citizen Engagement and the Learning Health System: Workshop Summary*. Edited by LeighAnne Olsen, Robert S. Saunders, and J. Michael McGinnis. Washington, DC: National Academies Press, 2011. doi:10.17226/12848.

——. *Treatment for Posttraumatic Stress Disorder in Military and Veteran Populations: Initial Assessment*. Washington, DC: National Academies Press, 2012. doi:10.17226/13364.

Ivany, Christopher G., Kelly W. Bickel, Tari Rangel, James Sarver, Joann Dinkel-Holzer, Dennis M. Sarmiento, and Charles W. Hoge. "Impact of a Service Line Management Model on Behavioral Health Care in the Military Health System." *Psychiatric Services* 70, no. 6 (2019): 522–25.

Jacobs, E. C. "PULHES, the Physical Profile Serial System." *United States Armed Forces Medical Journal* 4, no. 2 (February 1953): 235–41.

Jain, Anshu K., Jon M. Thompson, Scott M. Kelley, and Richard W. Schwartz. "Fundamentals of Service Lines and the Necessity of Physician Leaders." *Surgical Innovation* 13, no. 2 (2006): 136–44.

The Joint Commission. *Ambulatory Care Program: The Who, What, When, and Where's of Credentialing and Privileging*. Oakbrook Terrace, IL: Joint Commission, n.d. https://www.jointcommission.org/assets/1/6/AHC_who_what_when_and_where_credentialing_booklet.pdf.

——. *Revised Outcome Measures Standard for Behavioral Health Care*. R3 report, issue 13. Oakbrook Terrace, IL: Joint Commission, 2018.

Joynt, Karen E., and Ashish K. Jha. "Thirty-Day Readmissions—Truth and Consequences." *New England Journal of Medicine* 366, no. 15 (2012): 1366–69.

Kendrick, T., M. El-Gohary, B. Stuart, S. Gilbody, R. Churchill, L. Aiken, A. Bhattacharya, A. Gimson, A. L. Brütt, K. de Jong, and M. Moore. "Routine Use of Patient Reported Outcome Measures (PROMs) for Improving Treatment of Common Mental Health Disorders in Adults." *Cochrane Database of Systematic Reviews* 7 (2016).

Kim, Paul Y., Thomas W. Britt, Robert P. Klocko, Lyndon A. Riviere, and Amy B. Adler. "Stigma, Negative Attitudes about Treatment, and Utilization of Mental Health Care Among Soldiers." *Military Psychology*, 2011.

Kochan, Thomas A., John S. Carroll, Amy K. Glasmeier, Richard C. Larson, Anne Quaadgras, and Jayakanth Srinivasan. *PTSI Final Report Executive Summary: Transforming the Psychological Health System of Care in the US Military*. Cambridge, MA: Massachusetts Institute of Technology, 2016. https://dspace.mit.edu/handle/1721.1/102660.

Kripalani, Sunil, Cecelia N. Theobald, Beth Anctil, and Eduard E. Vasilevskis. "Reducing Hospital Readmission Rates: Current Strategies and Future Directions." *Annual Review of Medicine* 65, no. 1 (2014): 471–85.

Lewis, Byan. "New PTSD Program Answers Need." US Army, July 21, 2009. https://www.army.mil/article/24682.

Lineberry, Timothy W., and Stephen S. O'Connor. "Suicide in the US Army." *Mayo Clinic Proceedings* 87, no. 9 (2012): 872.

Linehan, Marsha M., Katherine Anne Comtois, Angela M. Murray, Milton Z. Brown, Robert J. Gallop, Heidi L. Heard, Kathryn E. Korslund, Darren A. Tutek, Sarah K. Reynolds, and Noam Lindenboim. "Two-Year Randomized Controlled Trial and Follow-up of Dialectical Behavior Therapy vs. Therapy by Experts for Suicidal Behaviors and Borderline Personality Disorder." *Archives of General Psychiatry* 63, no. 7 (2006): 757–66.

Lomas, Jonathan. "Diffusion, Dissemination, and Implementation: Who Should Do What?" *Annals of the New York Academy of Sciences* 703, no. 1 (1993): 226–37.

Lyons, John S., Michael T. O'Mahoney, Sheldon I. Miller, Janice Neme, Julie Kabat, and Fredrick Miller. "Predicting Readmission to the Psychiatric Hospital in a Managed Care Environment: Implications for Quality Indicators." *American Journal of Psychiatry* 154, no. 3 (1997): 337–40.

MaCurdy, Thomas, Jason Kerwin, Jonathan Gibbs, Eugene Lin, Carolyn Cotterman, Margaret O'Brien-Strain, Nick Theobald, and Frederick Thomas. *Evaluating the Functionality of the Symmetry ETG and Medstat MEG Software in Forming Episodes of Care Using Medicare Data.* Centers for Medicare and Medicaid Services (CMS). Burlingame, CA: Acumen, 2008.

Malish, Richard G., Anthony D. Arnett, and Ronald J. Place. "Returning to Duty from Temporary Disability in the U.S. Army: Observational Data and Commentary for Commanders, Providers, and Soldiers." *Military Medicine* 179, no. 11 (2014): 1190–97.

Maliwal, Neha. *Healthcare Analytics: Technologies and Global Markets.* BCC Market Research Report HLC187B. Wellesley, MA: BCC Publishing, 2017. https://www.bccresearch.com/market-research/healthcare/healthcare-analytics-technologies-markets-report.html.

Marmor, Theodore R., and Karyn C. Gill. "The Political and Economic Context of Mental Health Care in the United States." *Journal of Health Politics, Policy and Law* 14, no. 3 (1989): 459–75.

Maslach, Christina, and Julie Goldberg. "Prevention of Burnout: New Perspectives." *Applied and Preventive Psychology* 7, no. 1 (1998): 63–74.

Maslach, Christina, and Susan E. Jackson. "Patterns of Burnout among a National Sample of Public Contact Workers." *Journal of Health and Human Resources Administration* 7, no. 2 (1984): 189–212.

Maslach, Christina, Wilmar B. Schaufeli, and Michael P. Leiter. "Job Burnout." *Annual Review of Psychology* 52, no. 1 (2001): 397–422.

McIlvaine, Rob. "Chiarelli Says Research Continuing on 'Unseen Traumas.'" US Army, November 10, 2011. https://www.army.mil/article/69060/.

Mechanic, Robert E. "Opportunities and Challenges for Episode-Based Payment." *New England Journal of Medicine* 365, no. 9 (2011): 777–79.

Menninger, William C. *A Psychiatrist for a Troubled World: Selected Papers of William C. Menninger.* Vol. 2. Edited by Bernard H. Hall. New York: Viking Press, 1967.

Meslin, Eric M., Alessandro Blasimme, and Anne Cambon-Thomsen. "Mapping the Translational Science Policy 'Valley of Death.'" *Clinical and Translational Medicine* 2, no. 1 (2013): 14.

Meyer, Bjorn, Paul A. Pilkonis, Janice L. Krupnick, Matthew K. Egan, Samuel J. Simmens, and Stuart M. Sotsky. "Treatment Expectancies, Patient Alliance and Outcome: Further Analyses from the National Institute of Mental Health Treatment of Depression Collaborative Research Program." *Journal of Consulting and Clinical Psychology* 70, no. 4 (2002): 1051–55.

Michaelis, Björn, Ralf Stegmaier, and Karlheinz Sonntag. "Affective Commitment to Change and Innovation Implementation Behavior: The Role of Charismatic Leadership and

Employees' Trust in Top Management." *Journal of Change Management* 9, no. 4 (2009): 399–417.
——. "Shedding Light on Followers' Innovation Implementation Behavior: The Role of Transformational Leadership, Commitment to Change, and Climate for Initiative." *Journal of Managerial Psychology* 25, no. 4 (2010): 408–29.
Middleton, Allen, and Mike Dinneen. "Achieving the Quadruple Aim Focusing on Strategic Imperatives." Presentation at the Military Health System Conference, National Harbor, MD, January 24–27, 2011.
Miller, Alec L., Jill H. Rathus, and Marsha M. Linehan. *Dialectical Behavior Therapy with Suicidal Adolescents*. New York: Guilford Press, 2006.
Miller, Alec L., Jill H. Rathus, Marsha N. Linehan, Scott Wetzler, and Ellen Leigh. "Dialectical Behavior Therapy Adapted for Suicidal Adolescent." *Psychiatry and Behavioral Science* 3, no. 2 (1997).
Millikan, Amy M., Michael R. Bell, M. Shayne Gallaway, Maureen T. Lagana, Anthony L. Cox, and Michael G. Sweda. "An Epidemiologic Investigation of Homicides at Fort Carson, Colorado: Summary of Findings." *Military Medicine* 177, no. 4 (2012): 404–11.
Milliken, Charles S., Jennifer L. Auchterlonie, and Charles W. Hoge. "Longitudinal Assessment of Mental Health Problems among Active and Reserve Component Soldiers Returning from the Iraq War." *JAMA* 298, no. 18 (2007): 2141–48.
MIT Collaborative Initiatives. "Stroke Pathways." MIT Collaborative Initiatives, 2014. https://collaborative.mit.edu/projects/stroke-pathways.
Morris, David W., and Madhukar H. Trivedi. "Measurement-Based Care for Unipolar Depression." *Current Psychiatry Reports* 13, no. 6 (2011): 446–58.
National Institute of Mental Health. "Mental Illness." Last updated November 2020. https://www.nimh.nih.gov/health/statistics/mental-illness.shtml.
Nightingale, Deborah J., Wileana Glover, and Jayakanth Srinivasan. *Applying Lean to the Mental Health Services Enterprise: A Current State Analysis*. Cambridge, MA: Massachusetts Institute of Technology, 2011.
Office of the Surgeon General, US Army Medical Command. *Army Medicine Campaign Plan 2020*. Falls Church, VA: Office of the Surgeon General, 2013.
——. *Investigation of Homicides at Fort Carson, Colorado, November 2008–May 2009, Final Report*. Epidemiologic Consultation No. 14-HK-OB1U-09. Falls Church, VA: Office of the Surgeon General, 2009.
——. *Joint Mental Health Advisory Team 7 (J-MHAT 7) Operation Enduring Freedom 2010: Afghanistan (Redacted)*. Falls Church, VA: Office of the Surgeon General, 2010. https://ntrl.ntis.gov/NTRL/dashboard/searchResults/titleDetail/ADA543997.xhtml.
——. *MEDCOM MTF Enrollment, Access and Appointment Standards for all Uniformed Service Members, with Special Emphasis on Enhanced Access to Care for Specified Populations*. Policy 12-006. Falls Church, VA: Office of the Surgeon General, 2012.
——. "Memorandum: Guidance for the Behavioral Health Service Line (BHSL) Distribution MATRIX Tool (DMT)." Washington, DC: US Army, 2014.
——. "Memorandum: Interim MEDCOM Balanced Scorecard Strategy Map." Fort Sam Houston, TX: US Army, 2007.
——. *Mental Health Advisory Team (MHAT-III) Operation Iraqi Freedom 04-06 Final Report*. Washington, DC: Office of the Surgeon General, 2006. https://ntrl.ntis.gov/NTRL/dashboard/searchResults/titleDetail/PB2010104250.xhtml.
——. *Mental Health Advisory Team (MHAT) IV Operation Iraqi Freedom 05-07*. Washington, DC: Office of the Surgeon General, 2006. https://ntrl.ntis.gov/NTRL/dashboard/searchResults/titleDetail/PB2010103335.xhtml.

——. *Mental Health Advisory Team (MHAT) V Operation Iraqi Freedom 06-08: Iraq; Operation Enduring Freedom 8: Afghanistan*. Washington, DC: Office of the Surgeon General, 2008. https://ntrl.ntis.gov/NTRL/dashboard/searchResults/titleDetail/PB2010104247.xhtml.

——. *Mental Health Advisory Team (MHAT) 6 Operation Enduring Freedom 2009: Afghanistan*. Washington, DC: Office of the Surgeon General, 2009. https://ntrl.ntis.gov/NTRL/dashboard/searchResults/titleDetail/PB2010104248.xhtml.

——. *War Psychiatry*. Volume 4. Washington, DC: Office of the Surgeon General, 1995.

Olsen, Leigh Anne, Dara Aisner, and J. Michael McGinnis. "The Learning Healthcare System" Workshop Summary." *National Academies Press*, 2007.

Oslin, David W., Jennifer Ross, Steve Sayers, John Murphy, Vince Kane, and Ira R. Katz. "Screening, Assessment, and Management of Depression in VA Primary Care Clinics." *Journal of General Internal Medicine* 21, no. 1 (2006): 46–50.

Philipps, David. *Lethal Warriors: When the New Band of Brothers Came Home*. New York: St. Martin's Press, 2010.

Pomerantz, Andrew S., Lisa K. Kearney, Laura O. Wray, Edward P. Post, and John F. McCarthy. "Mental Health Services in the Medical Home in the Department of Veterans Affairs: Factors for Successful Integration." *Psychological Services* 11, no. 3 (2014): 243–53.

Porter, Michael E., and Thomas H. Lee. "The Strategy That Will Fix Health Care." *Harvard Business Review* 91, no. 10 (2013): 1–19.

Porter, Rebecca. "The Army Comprehensive Behavioral Health System of Care (CBHSOC) Campaign Plan." Presentation at the Military Health System Conference, National Harbor, MD, January 24–27, 2011. https://ntrl.ntis.gov/NTRL/dashboard/searchResults/titleDetail/ADA556255.xhtml.

Prine, Carl. "Army's Mental Health Programs Swamped, Understaffed." *Pittsburgh Tribune-Gazette*, February 7, 2011. https://archive.triblive.com/news/armys-mental-health-programs-swamped-understaffed-2/.

Quartana, Phillip J., Joshua E. Wilk, Jeffrey L. Thomas, Robert M. Bray, Kristine L. Rae Olmsted, Janice M. Brown, Jason Williams, Paul Y. Kim, Kristina Clarke-Walper, and Charles W. Hoge. "Trends in Mental Health Services Utilization and Stigma in US Soldiers from 2002 to 2011." *American Journal of Public Health* 104, no. 9 (2014): 1671–79.

Rathus, Jill H., and Alec L. Miller. "Dialectical Behavior Therapy Adapted for Suicidal Adolescents." *Suicide and Life-Threatening Behavior* 32, no. 2 (2002): 146–57.

Reason, James. "Human Error: Models and Management." *BMJ* 320, no. 7237 (2000): 768–70.

Reza, Virginia. "Chief Says Army Needs to Replicate Bliss PTSD Program." US Army, July 18, 2008. https://www.army.mil/article/11001/.

Rieckhoff, Paul. "Dole-Shalala Commission Report: Walter Reed Was Just the Beginning." *Huffington Post*, July 26, 2007. Updated May 25, 2011. https://www.huffpost.com/entry/doleshalala-commission-re_b_57879.

Roberts, Chris. "Fort Bliss' Restoration and Resilience Center Offers War-Damaged Minds Solace, Treatment." *El Paso Times*, March 30, 2009. https://www.army.mil/article/18943/.

Rosen, Allison B., Eli Liebman, Ana Aizcorbe, and M. Cutler. *Comparing Commercial Systems for Characterizing Episodes of Care*. BEA Working Paper no. WP2012-7. Washington, DC: Bureau of Economic Analysis, 2012. https://econpapers.repec.org/paper/beawpaper/0085.htm.

Rubenstein, Lisa V., Edmund F. Chaney, Scott Ober, Bradford Felker, Scott E. Sherman, Andy Lanto, and Susan Vivell. "Using Evidence-Based Quality Improvement Methods for Translating Depression Collaborative Care Research into Practice." *Families, Systems, and Health* 28, no. 2 (2010): 91–113.

Rubenstein, Lisa V., and Jacqueline Pugh. "Strategies for Promoting Organizational and Practice Change by Advancing Implementation Research." *Journal of General Internal Medicine* 21, no. 2 (2006): S58.

Salmon, T. W., and N. Fenton. "In the American Expeditionary Forces [Section 2]." *Neuropsychiatry* 10 (1929).

Scott, Kelli, and Cara C. Lewis. "Using Measurement-Based Care to Enhance Any Treatment." *Cognitive and Behavioral Practice* 22, no. 1 (2015): 49–59.

Scott, Shane P. "Network Governance for the Provision of Behavioral Health Services to the US Army." MS thesis, Massachusetts Institute of Technology, 2012.

Shenbergerhess, Ashley. "Senior Military Leader's Share Experiences in Mental Health." *US Army*, April 22, 2019. https://www.army.mil/article/220665/senior_military_leaders_share_experiences_in_mental_health.

Shephard, Ben. *A War of Nerves: Soldiers and Psychiatrists in the Twentieth Century*. Cambridge: Harvard University Press, 2001.

Smith, Christopher L. "The Fort Carson Murder Spree." *Rolling Stone*, November 12, 2009. https://www.rollingstone.com/politics/politics-news/the-fort-carson-murder-spree-200137/.

Sontag, Deborah, and Lizette Alvarez. "Iraq Veterans Leave a Trail of Death and Heartbreak in U.S." *New York Times*, January 13, 2008. https://www.nytimes.com/2008/01/13/world/americas/13iht-vets.1.9171147.html.

Spitzer, Robert L., Kurt Kroenke, Janet B. W. Williams, and the Patient Health Questionnaire Primary Care Study Group. "Validation and Utility of a Self-Report Version of PRIME-MD: PHQ Primary Care Study." *JAMA* 282, no. 18 (1999): 1737–44.

Srinivasan, Jayakanth, John S. Carroll, and Julia M. DiBenigno. "US Army: Transformation to a Behavioral Health System of Care." Chapter 2 of *PTSI Report: Transforming the Psychological Health System of Care in the US Military*. Cambridge, MA: Massachusetts Institute of Technology, 2016. https://dspace.mit.edu/handle/1721.1/102565.

Srinivasan, Jayakanth, Julia DiBenigno, and John S. Carroll. "Transformation of the US Army Behavioral Health System of Care: An Organizational Analysis Using the Three Lenses." *Journal of Organizational Behavior Education* 10, no. 1 (2017): 5–28.

Stahl, Stephen M. "Crisis in Army Psychopharmacology and Mental Health Care at Fort Hood." *CNS Spectrums* 14, no. 12 (2009): 677–84.

Substance Abuse and Mental Health Services Administration. *Metrics and Quality Measures for Behavioral Health Clinics Technical Specifications and Resource Manual*. Vol. 1. Washington, DC: Substance Abuse and Mental Health Services Administration, 2016. https://www.samhsa.gov/section-223/quality-measures.

Swan, Jacky, Susan Newell, and Davide Nicolini. *Mobilizing Knowledge in Health Care: Challenges for Management and Organization*. Oxford: Oxford University Press, 2016.

Szabo, Liz. "Cost of Not Caring: Nowhere to Go." *USA Today*, May 12, 2014. https://www.usatoday.com/story/news/nation/2014/05/12/mental-health-system-crisis/7746535/.

Tanielian, Terri, and Lisa H. Jaycox, eds. *Invisible Wounds of War: Psychological and Cognitive Injuries, Their Consequences, and Services to Assist Recovery*. Santa Monica, CA: RAND Corporation, 2008. https://www.rand.org/pubs/monographs/MG720.html.

Thomas, Fred, Craig Caplan, Jesse M. Levy, Marty Cohen, James Leonard, Todd Caldis, and Curt Mueller. "Clinician Feedback on Using Episode Groupers with Medicare Claims Data." *Health Care Financing Review* 31, no. 1 (2009): 1–11.

Thornicroft, Graham, Michele Tansella, and Ann Law. "Steps, Challenges and Lessons in Developing Community Mental Health Care." *World Psychiatry* 7, no. 2 (2008): 87–92.

Tucker, Anita L., and Amy C. Edmondson. "Why Hospitals Don't Learn from Failures: Organizational and Psychological Dynamics That Inhibit System Change." *California Management Review* 45, no. 2 (2003): 55–72.

US Army Medical Command. "Army Substance Use Disorder Clinical Care." *Stand To!*, September 21, 2016. https://www.army.mil/standto/archive_2016-09-21/.

——. *Behavioral Health Business Practice and Coding Guidelines.* 2nd ed. Falls Church, VA: Department of the Army, 2017.

——. *Embedded Behavioral Health Operations Manual.* Falls Church, VA: Department of the Army, 2014.

——. "Embedded Behavioral Health Team (EBHT) Implementation." Operational Order 12–63. Falls Church, VA: Department of the Army, 2012.

——. "Medical Evaluation Board Phase Implementation Guidance." Annex O, Operations Order 12–31. Falls Church, VA: Department of the Army, 2012.

US Army Public Health Command. *Surveillance of Suicidal Behavior, January through December 2013.* Public Health Report No. S.0008057-13. Aberdeen Proving Ground, MD: US Army Public Health Command, 2015. http://www.dtic.mil/docs/citations/ADA619599.

US Army Public Health Command (Provisional). *Program Consultation (PROCON) Part I: Retrospective Evaluation of a Mobile Behavioral Health Service in Garrison Fort Carson, Colorado.* 23-KM-0C93-10. Aberdeen Proving Ground, MD: US Army Public Health Command, 2010.

US Congress. Senate. *Department of Defense Appropriations for Fiscal Year 2012: Hearing before the Subcommittee of the Committee on Appropriations.* 111th Cong., 2nd sess., April 6, 2011. Statement of Lieutenant General Eric. B. Schoomaker. https://www.appropriations.senate.gov/imo/media/doc/hearings/04_06_2011%20Defense%20DoD%20Health%20Programs%20GPO%20Record.pdf.

US Department of Defense. *Mental Health Evaluations of Members of the Armed Services.* DoD Instruction 6490.04. Washington, DC: US Department of Defense, 2013. http://www.esd.whs.mil/Portals/54/Documents/DD/issuances/dodi/649004p.pdf.

U.S. Department of Defense, Assistant Secretary of Defense for Health Affairs. *Tricare Policy for Access to Care.* Policy 11-005. February 23, 2011.

US Department of Defense, Task Force on Mental Health. *An Achievable Vision: Report of the Department of Defense Task Force on Mental Health.* Falls Church, VA: Defense Health Board, 2007. https://apps.dtic.mil/dtic/tr/fulltext/u2/a469411.pdf.

US Department of Defense, Task Force on Military Health System Governance. *Final Report.* Vol. 1. Washington, DC: US Department of Defense, 2011.

US Department of the Army. *Army 2020: Generating Health and Discipline in the Force Ahead of Strategic Reset.* Washington, DC: Department of the Army, 2012. https://www.army.mil/e2/c/downloads/235822.pdf.

——. *Army Health Promotion Risk Reduction Suicide Prevention Report 2010.* Washington, DC: Department of the Army, 2010. https://preventsuicide.army.mil/docs/Commanders%20Tool%20Kit/HPRRSP_Report_2010_v00.pdf.

——. *Leader's Manual for Combat Stress Control.* FM 22–51. Washington, DC: Department of the Army, 1994.

US Department of the Army Headquarters. "Army Implementation of Behavioral Health System of Care (BHSOC) Embedded Behavioral Health (EBH)." ALARACT HQDA EXORD 236–12. Washington, DC: Department of the Army, 2012.

——. "Vice Chief of Staff of the Army (VCSA) Sends on Protected Health Information (PHI)." ALARACT 160/2/10. Washington, DC: Department of the Army, 2012.

US Department of Veterans Affairs, Office of the Inspector General. *Audit of Alleged Manipulation of Waiting Times in Veterans Integrated Service Network 3*. Washington, DC: Department of Veterans Affairs, 2008. https://www.va.gov/oig/52/reports/2008/VAOIG-07-03505-129.pdf.

US Government Accountability Office. *Defense Health Care: Additional Information Needed about Mental Health Provider Staffing Need*. GAO-15-184. Washington, DC: US Government Accountability Office, 2015. https://www.gao.gov/products/GAO-15-184.

——. *Defense Health Care: DOD Should Demonstrate How Its Plan to Transfer the Administration of Military Treatment Facilities Will Improve Efficiency*. GAO-19-53. Washington, DC: US Government Accountability Office, 2018. https://www.gao.gov/products/gao-19-53.

——. *Defense Health: Coordinating Authority Needed for Psychological Health and Traumatic Brain Injury Activities*. GAO-12-154. Washington, DC: US Government Accountability Office, 2012. https://www.gao.gov/products/GAO-12-154.

US Health Resources & Service Administration. "What is Shortage Designation?" https://bhw.hrsa.gov/workforce-shortage-areas/shortage-designation.

US President's Commission on Care for America's Returning Wounded Warriors. *Serve, Support, Simplify: Report of the President's Commission on Care for America's Returning Wounded Warriors*. Washington, DC: President's Commission on Care for America's Returning Wounded Warriors, 2007. https://www.loc.gov/item/2007467172/.

Valenstein, Marcia, David A. Adler, Jeffery Berlant, Lisa B. Dixon, Rebecca A. Dulit, Beth Goldman, Ann Hackman, David W. Oslin, Samuel G. Siris, and William A. Sonis. "Implementing Standardized Assessments in Clinical Care: Now's the Time." *Psychiatric Services* 60, no. 10 (2009): 1372–75.

Vedantam, Shankar. "A Political Debate on Stress Disorder." *Washington Post*, December 27, 2005. https://www.washingtonpost.com/archive/politics/2005/12/27/a-political-debate-on-stress-disorder/115a753d-5dac-41a0-b9fe-9fe457fb5320/.

Veterans Health Administration. *VHA Handbook 1160.01: Uniform Mental Health Services in VA Medical Centers and Clinics*. Washington, DC: Department of Veterans Affairs, 2008. https://www.va.gov/vhapublications/ViewPublication.asp?pub_ID=1762.

Von Hippel, Eric, and Georg von Krogh. "CROSSROADS—Identifying Viable 'Need–Solution Pairs': Problem Solving without Problem Formulation." *Organization Science* 27, no. 1 (2016): 207–21.

Watts, Bradley V., Brian Shiner, Andrew Pomerantz, Patricia Stender, and William B. Weeks. "Outcomes of a Quality Improvement Project Integrating Mental Health into Primary Care." *Quality and Safety in Health Care* 16, no. 5 (2007): 378–81.

Weber, Eve, and David K. Weber. "Deployment Limiting Mental Health Conditions in US Military Personnel Deployed to Combat Theaters: Predictors of Theater Mental Health Evacuation." *Journal of Psychology and Clinical Psychiatry* 2, no. 4 (2015).

Weinick, Robin M., Ellen Burke Beckjord, Carrie M. Farmer, Laurie T. Martin, Emily M. Gillen, Joie D. Acosta, Michael P. Fisher, Jeffrey Garnett, Gabriella C. Gonzalez, Todd C. Helmus, Lisa H. Jaycox, Kerry Reynolds, Nicholas Salcedo, and Deborah M. Scharf. *Programs Addressing Psychological Health and Traumatic Brain Injury among U.S. Military Servicemembers and Their Families*. Santa Monica, CA: RAND Corporation, 2011. https://www.rand.org/pubs/technical_reports/TR950.html.

Weist, Mark D. "Expanded School Mental Health Services: A National Movement in Progress." In *Advances in Clinical Child Psychology*, edited by T. H. Ollendick and R. J. Prinz, 319–52. Boston: Springer, 1997.

Weist, Mark D., Nancy A. Lever, Catherine P. Bradshaw, and Julie Sarno Owens. "Further Advancing the Field of School Mental Health." In *Handbook of School Mental*

Health, edited by M. Weist, N. Lever, C. Bradshaw, and J. Owens, 1–14. New York: Springer, 2014.

Zeiss, Antonette M., and Bradley E. Karlin. "Integrating Mental Health and Primary Care Services in the Department of Veterans Affairs Health Care System." *Journal of Clinical Psychology in Medical Settings* 15, no. 1 (2008): 73–78.

Index

Page numbers in italics indicate figures; those with a *t* indicate tables.